ABC of
Clinical Communication

D1587026

WITHDRAWN
FROM LIBRARY
BRITISH MEDICAL ASSOCIATION

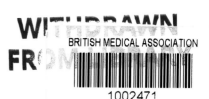

1002471

ABC series

An outstanding collection of resources for everyone in primary care

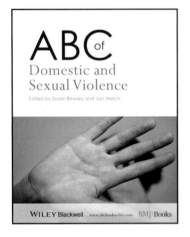
ABC of
Domestic and
Sexual Violence
Edited by Susan Bewley and Jan Welch
WILEY Blackwell   www.abcbookseries.com   BMJ|Books

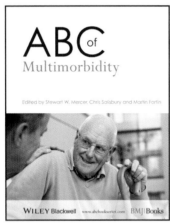
ABC of
Multimorbidity
Edited by Stewart W. Mercer, Chris Salisbury and Martin Fortin
WILEY Blackwell   www.abcbookseries.com   BMJ|Books

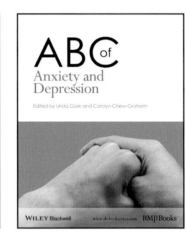
ABC of
Anxiety and
Depression
Edited by Linda Gask and Carolyn Chew-Graham
WILEY Blackwell   www.abcbookseries.com   BMJ|Books

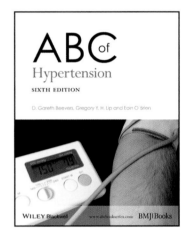
ABC of
Hypertension
SIXTH EDITION
D. Gareth Beevers, Gregory Y. H. Lip and Eoin O'Brien
WILEY Blackwell   www.abcbookseries.com   BMJ|Books

The *ABC* Series contains a wealth of indispensable resources for GPs, GP registrars, junior doctors, and all those in primary care

- **Highly illustrated, informative, and practical**

- **Covers the symptoms, investigations, and treatment and management of conditions presenting in daily practice**

- **Full colour photographs and illustrations aid diagnosis and patient understanding**

For more information on all books in the ABC series, including links to further information, references and links to the latest official guidelines, please visit:

www.abcbookseries.com

BMJ|Books

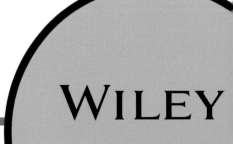
WILEY

ABC of

Clinical Communication

EDITED BY

Nicola Cooper, MBChB, FAcadMEd, FRCPE, FRACP
Consultant Physician and Honorary Clinical Associate Professor
Derby Teaching Hospitals NHS Foundation Trust
Derby, UK

John Frain, MBChB, MSc, FRCGP, DGM, DCH, DRCOG, PGDipCard
Director of Clinical Skills
Division of Medical Sciences and Graduate Entry Medicine
University of Nottingham
Nottingham, UK

WILEY Blackwell

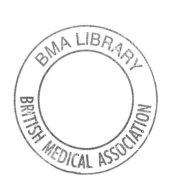

This edition first published 2018
© 2018 John Wiley & Sons Ltd

All rights reserved. No part of this publication may be reproduced, stored in a retrieval system, or transmitted, in any form or by any means, electronic, mechanical, photocopying, recording or otherwise, except as permitted by law. Advice on how to obtain permission to reuse material from this title is available at http://www.wiley.com/go/permissions.

The right of Nicola Cooper and John Frain to be identified as the authors of the editorial material in this work has been asserted in accordance with law.

Registered Offices
John Wiley & Sons, Inc., 111 River Street, Hoboken, NJ 07030, USA
John Wiley & Sons Ltd, The Atrium, Southern Gate, Chichester, West Sussex, PO19 8SQ, UK

Editorial Office
9600 Garsington Road, Oxford, OX4 2DQ, UK

For details of our global editorial offices, customer services, and more information about Wiley products visit us at www.wiley.com.

Wiley also publishes its books in a variety of electronic formats and by print-on-demand. Some content that appears in standard print versions of this book may not be available in other formats.

Limit of Liability/Disclaimer of Warranty
In view of ongoing research, equipment modifications, changes in governmental regulations, and the constant flow of information relating to the use of experimental reagents, equipment, and devices, the reader is urged to review and evaluate the information provided in the package insert or instructions for each chemical, piece of equipment, reagent, or device for, among other things, any changes in the instructions or indication of usage and for added warnings and precautions. While the publisher and authors have used their best efforts in preparing this work, they make no representations or warranties with respect to the accuracy or completeness of the contents of this work and specifically disclaim all warranties, including without limitation any implied warranties of merchantability or fitness for a particular purpose. No warranty may be created or extended by sales representatives, written sales materials or promotional statements for this work. The fact that an organization, website, or product is referred to in this work as a citation and/or potential source of further information does not mean that the publisher and authors endorse the information or services the organization, website, or product may provide or recommendations it may make. This work is sold with the understanding that the publisher is not engaged in rendering professional services. The advice and strategies contained herein may not be suitable for your situation. You should consult with a specialist where appropriate. Further, readers should be aware that websites listed in this work may have changed or disappeared between when this work was written and when it is read. Neither the publisher nor authors shall be liable for any loss of profit or any other commercial damages, including but not limited to special, incidental, consequential, or other damages.

Library of Congress Cataloging-in-Publication Data
Names: Cooper, Nicola, editor. | Frain, John (John Patrick James), editor.
Title: ABC of clinical communication / edited by Nicola Cooper, John Frain.
Description: Hoboken, NJ : Wiley, [2018] | Series: ABC series | Includes bibliographical references and index. |
Identifiers: LCCN 2017023660 (print) | LCCN 2017024788 (ebook) | ISBN 9781119246978 (pdf) |
  ISBN 9781119247005 (epub) | ISBN 9781119246985 (pbk.)
Subjects: | MESH: Professional-Patient Relations | Communication | Clinical Medicine
Classification: LCC R727.3 (ebook) | LCC R727.3 (print) | NLM W 62 | DDC 610.69/6–dc23
LC record available at https://lccn.loc.gov/2017023660

Cover Design: Wiley
Cover Image: © Clarissa Leahy/Gettyimages

Set in 9.25/12pt Minion by SPi Global, Pondicherry, India
Printed and bound in Singapore by Markono Print Media Pte Ltd

10 9 8 7 6 5 4 3 2 1

Contents

Preface

Good clinical communication is essential for safe patient care. Clinical communication occurs within the patient encounter, but also through information flow within and between clinical teams. Issues around communication account for the majority of complaints about patient care.

The last quarter of a century has seen the establishment of an evidence base for good communication skills and the teaching and assessment of it. We are now better placed to identify and to demonstrate the qualities required for effective communication with the range of patients and professionals encountered in clinical practice. Communication is a core part of curricula within medical schools. Students trained in the early days of these programmes are now practitioners and teachers themselves, meaning the practice and role-modelling of these skills are gradually increasing.

This book is intended as a reference for healthcare students and practitioners, either as part of a communication skills course or for personal study. Issues around clinical communication relate to skills required within the consultation, for communication within and between teams, in medical records and during handover.

Clinical communication concerns not only establishing rapport with patients and ensuring patient satisfaction with the encounter on a human level – it also means actively listening to patients and understanding their experience and perspective on the anatomical and physiological changes that may constitute pathology and disease. Detailed gathering of hard clinical data reduces the risk of diagnostic error and leads to better treatment and management decisions.

Although this book inevitably reflects our own work in the UK's National Health Service, we are pleased to have brought together a range of international authors, all of whom are recognised experts in their fields. It has been a pleasure to edit this book and in the process to understand better the development of our own communication with patients, students and colleagues. We hope you enjoy and learn from it.

Nicola Cooper & John Frain
January 2017

Contributors

Magdy Abdalla, MBCHB, FRCSI, DRCOG, FRCGP, MMedSci

GP Teaching Fellow, Division of Medical Sciences and Graduate Entry Medicine
University of Nottingham, Nottingham, UK

Nivedita Aswani, MBChB, MRCPCH

Consultant Paediatrician, Lead for Paediatric Diabetes, Derbyshire Children's Hospital, Derby, UK

Phyllis Butow, BA (Hons), DipEd, MClinPsych, MPH, PhD

Psycho-Oncology Cooperative Research Group (PoCoG) & Centre for Medical Psychology and Evidence-based Decision-making, School of Psychology
Surgical Outcomes Research Centre (SoURCE), Institute of Surgery, University of Sydney, Sydney, Australia

Gillian B. Clack, PhD(Lond)

Former Honorary Senior Lecturer, Division of Medical Education, King's College London, London, UK

Josephine Clayton, MBBS (Hons), PhD, FRACP, FAChPM

HammondCare Palliative and Supportive Care Service, Greenwich Hospital, Greenwich, Sydney;
Kolling Institute, Northern Clinical School, Faculty of Medicine, University of Sydney, Sydney, Australia

Nicola Cooper, MBChB, FAcadMEd, FRCPE, FRACP

Consultant Physician and Honorary Clinical Associate Professor, Derby Teaching Hospitals NHS Foundation Trust, Derby, UK

Vanessa Cox, MBChB, MRCPCH

Consultant Paediatrician, Derbyshire Children's Hospital, Derby, UK

Alison Cracknell, MBChB, FRCP, PGCert

Consultant Physician, Honorary Clinical Associate Professor and Patient Safety Lead, The Leeds Teaching Hospitals NHS Trust, Leeds, UK

John Frain, MBChB, MSc, FRCGP, DGM, DCH, DRCOG, PGDipCard

Director of Clinical Skills, Division of Medical Sciences and Graduate Entry Medicine, University of Nottingham, Nottingham, UK

Jonathan Silverman, BA, BM. BCh, FRCGP, FAcadMEd

President of the European Association for Communication in Healthcare, Honorary Visiting Senior Fellow, School of Clinical Medicine, University of Cambridge, Cambridge, UK

Lee Smith, BA, PGDip, MA, MA, RMN

Mental Health Nurse Specialist, Derbyshire Healthcare NHS Foundation Trust, Derby, UK

Nigel D.C. Sturrock, BMSc, MBChB, MSc, MD, FRCP

Executive Medical Director, Derby Teaching Hospitals NHS Foundation Trust, Derby, UK

Julia Surridge, MBBS, DRCOG, DCH, MRCPCH, PGCert (Med Ed)

Paediatric Emergency Medicine Consultant, Derbyshire Children's Hospital, Derby, UK

Adam Walczak, BPsych (Hons), PhD

Youth Cancer Services & Clinical Trials Division, CanTeen Australia, Sydney, Australia

Andy Wearn, MBChB, MMedSc, MRCGP

Director, Clinical Skills Centre, Faculty of Medical & Health Sciences, The University of Auckland, Auckland, New Zealand

CHAPTER 1

Why Clinical Communication Matters

John Frain

University of Nottingham, Nottingham, UK

OVERVIEW

- The clinical interview is essential in collecting information about a patient and reducing diagnostic error.
- There is an evidence base for the skills that best facilitate collection of both the biomedical and psychosocial content of the patient's story.
- Good clinical communication underpins patient-centred care.
- Health professionals require continuing training in clinical communication in all its forms.
- Efficient information flow within the healthcare team is an essential component of patient safety.
- Respect for patients and colleagues is a prerequisite for effective clinical communication.

Clinical communication – a historical perspective

In the absence of defined physical examination methods and investigations, such as blood tests and imaging, interviewing the patient was the mainstay of diagnosing illness and managing disease. While we know little of the format of the doctor–patient encounter prior to the nineteenth century, *listening* was a virtue associated with the competent doctor. The doctor relied on the patient's description of symptoms to make a diagnosis. As only wealthier members of society could afford the services of a doctor, good communication skills were rewarded with greater employment. The apprenticeship model of medical training led to the role-modelling of these skills by senior doctors. While the doctor–patient relationship has evolved since then (see Figure 1.1), the 'history' remains the most important means of making a diagnosis.

Improving knowledge of anatomy, physiology and the pathological basis of disease during the 1800s contributed to a structured clinical method consisting of a structured history and physical examination (see Box 1.1). William Osler, sometimes described as 'the father of modern medicine', took students from the lecture theatre to the patient's bedside so that students could talk to patients about their experience of disease and physically examine them for signs of the illness.

Even in an era of rapid change in the scientific basis of medicine, Osler's maxim to his students was: '*Listen to your patient; he is telling you the diagnosis.*' In modern times, the history alone accounts for around 80% of diagnoses. Strikingly, increasing availability of diagnostic technology (e.g. laboratory tests and imaging) has not substantially altered this percentage.

It is worth considering what the healthcare professional wishes to derive from the patient interview or encounter. The purpose is to:

- Correctly diagnose the patient's illness.
- Avoid diagnostic error.
- Give the patient effective and appropriate treatment.
- Achieve the patient's adherence to treatment.
- Cure or mitigate the effect of the illness.
- Improve the patient's health status.
- Communicate care, concern and empathy.

Early studies of the consultation correlated the quality of the interview directly with the quality of clinical data collected (see 'Further resources'). An open-ended approach with the intention of allowing patients to identify problems of concern identified those problems well. The failure of professionals to allow patients to complete an opening statement during the consultation and an over-controlling approach (e.g. using closed questions) directly reduced the quality of information.

Poor-quality information results in a predisposition to diagnostic error, and the term 'clinical hypocompetence' has been used to describe this (see Box 1.2). While a biomedical perspective has contributed to improvements in diagnosis, the use of a solely biomedical approach risks being reductionist as it fails to take account of the patient's own experience, context and wishes. The power imbalance between the 'all-knowing' professional and the passive patient contributes to poorer outcomes. The post-war era saw the development of societal concepts such as greater self-determination, autonomy, gender rights and equality. This influenced healthcare as well, with the result of the model of the consultation we have today (see Chapter 2).

ABC of Clinical Communication, First Edition. Edited by Nicola Cooper and John Frain.
© 2018 John Wiley & Sons Ltd. Published 2018 by John Wiley & Sons Ltd.

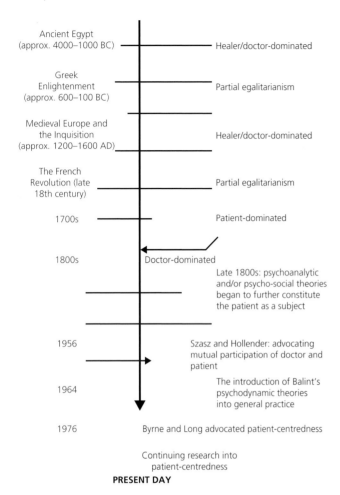

Figure 1.1 Evolution of the doctor–patient relationship. *Source*: Kaba and Sooriakumararan (2007). Reproduced with permission of Elsevier.

Box 1.1 **The traditional model of a structured patient history**

- Demographics
- Presenting problem(s)
- History of presenting problem(s)
- Past medical history
- Systems enquiry
- Family history
- Medications and allergies
- Social history

Source: Adapted from Stoeckle and Billings (1987). Reproduced with permission of Springer.

Even for the same illness, no two patients are going to give identical stories. Each will have a different experience of their symptoms and different concerns about their significance. Obeying Osler's maxim to *listen* requires seeing the patient's perspective and their own unique experience. If we needed to update Osler to make this clearer, we might say: '*Listen to your patient and see the illness through his eyes; he is telling you the diagnosis.*'

Box 1.2 **Clinical hypocompetence in the medical interview**

Physician-engendered defects in the interview are due to one or a combination of:
- Lack of therapeutic intent
- Inattention to primary data (symptoms)
- A high control style
- An incomplete database usually omitting patient-centred data and active problems other than the present illness
- A thoughtless interview in which the physician fails to formulate needed working hypotheses

Source: Adapted from Platt and McMath (1979). Reproduced with permission of American College of Physicians.

The emergence of a bio-psychosocial-cultural model placed emphasis not only on *what was the matter with the patient* but also, as Engel (1977) famously described, *what mattered to the patient*. This evolved further into one that enabled patients to fulfil their potential and ultimately into 'patient-centred medicine' in which the patient has to be understood as a unique human being. This approach has been endorsed by patients and professional and regulatory bodies across the world and much research has explored the factors influencing patient-centredness (see Figure 1.2).

Patient-centred care entails involvement in discussion of treatment options and decision-making, as well as sharing of information, including records (see Chapter 4). Shared decision-making improves patient and professional satisfaction with the consultation. It involves a common acceptance of the problem, discussion of the available management options, including their benefits and risks, eliciting the patient's own views and preferences for these options and then agreeing on a management plan.

In some respects, we have proceeded forward to the past as the evidence supports the wisdom of Osler's advice. Research has identified the skills that best determine important biomedical and psychosocial data and thus facilitate diagnosis. Over the last 40 years we have developed an evidence base for clinical communication associated with higher patient satisfaction. Several consultation models have been developed which form the basis of undergraduate and postgraduate training (see Box 1.3). We consider one of these models in Chapter 2. Barriers to its successful implementation include a continuing strong emphasis on the biomedical perspective with its doctor-centredness, time pressures and lack of ongoing appropriate training.

Educational interventions to teach good communication skills have been evaluated and accepted as good practice. All UK medical schools now provide training in communication. The use of simulated patients and models of feedback are also accepted as the norm in many training programmes. Teaching clinical communication is discussed in more detail in Chapter 10. The European Association for Communication in Healthcare has defined the learning objectives in a proposed core curriculum across all the health professions (Box 1.4).

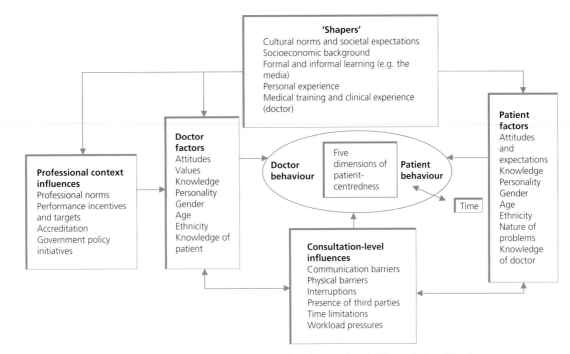

Figure 1.2 Factors influencing patient-centredness. *Source*: Mead and Bower (2000). Reproduced with permission of Elsevier.

Box 1.3 **Models of the consultation**

Established models include:
- Patient-centred clinical method (Brown *et al.*, 1986)
- Three function model (Bird & Cohen-Cole, 1990)
- E4 model (Keller & Carroll, 1994)
- Calgary-Cambridge guide (Silverman *et al.*, 1998)
- Patient-centred interviewing (Smith *et al.*, 2000; Fortin *et al.*, 2012)
- Four habits (Frankel & Stein, 2001)
- SEGUE framework (Makoul, 2001)

Source: Adapted from Brown *et al.* (2016). Reproduced with permission of Wiley.

Box 1.4 **Domains for a health professions core curriculum: objectives for undergraduate education in health care professions.**

- Communicating with patients
  - Core skills
  - Shaping of relationship
  - Patient's perspective and health beliefs
  - Information-sharing
  - Reasoning and decision-making
  - Dealing with uncertainty
- Intra- and interpersonal communication (professionalism and reflection)
  - Communication with self and others
  - Dealing with errors and uncertainty
- Communication in health care team (professional communication)
  - Teamwork and professional communication
  - Leadership
  - Professional communication and management

Source: Adapted from the European consensus. Reproduced with permission of Elsevier.

Effect of communication on patient outcomes

Improved interviewing, information-sharing and shared decision-making contribute to improved patient outcomes, particularly in chronic disease. There are reduced levels of patient discomfort and concern.

Patients perceive communication within the interview as a marker of quality. It is related to patient satisfaction, adherence to treatment, litigation, quality of data collection, patterns of use of services and clinical outcomes. Those behaviours associated with higher patient satisfaction are displayed in Figure 1.3.

Much has been achieved in the last 30–40 years and improvements in clinical communication are being implemented worldwide. Nonetheless, there remain a series of challenges if the actuality of patient-centred care is to be developed further. In addition to identifying relevant skills and factors affecting patient-centredness, research has also identified the adverse impacts on patient and staff well-being of poor communication. Each of these provides significant challenges for health services in the twenty-first century (see Box 1.5)

Training and feedback

Communication is one of the health professional's core skills. Patients place great value on quality of communication. To fulfil Osler's maxim, students need to be observed practising integration of both biomedical and psychosocial perspectives in the

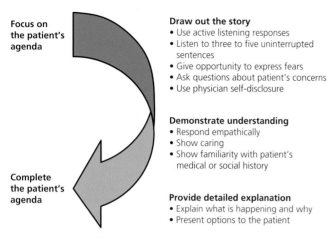

Draw out the story
- Use active listening responses
- Listen to three to five uninterrupted sentences
- Give opportunity to express fears
- Ask questions about patient's concerns
- Use physician self-disclosure

Demonstrate understanding
- Respond empathically
- Show caring
- Show familiarity with patient's medical or social history

Provide detailed explanation
- Explain what is happening and why
- Present options to the patient

Figure 1.3 Model of behaviours linked to higher patient satisfaction. *Source*: Tallman *et al.* Reproduced with permission of *Permanente Journal*.

Box 1.5 **Impact of poor communication in healthcare**

Poor communication in healthcare has an impact on the following aspects of patient care:
- Diagnostic accuracy
- Adherence to treatment
- Patient satisfaction
- Patient safety
- Team satisfaction
- Malpractice risk

---

consultation. While pre-qualification training includes communication, it is relatively rare for postgraduate trainees to receive instruction once qualified. While there is emphasis on improving one's knowledge after qualification, there exists little opportunity for direct observation and feedback on existing skills or the acquisition of new communication skills. Health professionals may not realise the possibility or need to improve their communication skills post-qualification. There is too often the assumption that these skills will automatically improve through exposure and experience, even though qualified health professionals are responsible for more complex communication tasks such as shared decision-making or breaking bad news, for which they may have had limited training as students. Continuing professional development and reflection on communication skills should not be dependent solely on receipt of adverse feedback or need for remediation. A core 'curriculum' for reflection on personal communication skills for significant events, appraisal or relicensing is suggested in Box 1.6. Clinical communication in more complex consultations is covered in Chapters 7–9.

It is in the interest of a healthcare provider to ensure there is development of clinical communication skills among its workforce. System-wide, relationship-centred training has a measurable impact on patient satisfaction scores. A further benefit is improved physician empathy, self-efficacy and reduced physician burnout. Short-term training (i.e. < 10 hours) is as successful as longer training. Courses can involve video or direct observation, debrief and feedback and group work involving role-play. Organisation-wide

---

Box 1.6 **Domains for reflection in advanced clinical communication**

- Responding to and managing own emotions
- Opportunistic promotion of health
- Managing uncertainty
- Shared decision-making
- Enabling self-care
- Responding to a complaint
- Candour and disclosure of medical error
- Communication within a multidisciplinary team

---

programmes of clinical communication training are effective when there is adherence to a single model, strong leadership and role-modelling, and outcomes include satisfaction of the professionals in training as well.

Communication between professionals

Clinical communication is not just about clinician and patient. Ineffective communication within and between teams contributes to over two-thirds of clinical errors. Healthcare professionals require skills not only to elicit clinical data in each encounter with a patient but also to efficiently convey this information to fellow professionals. Shared records can assist here (e.g. in maternity, child development, heart failure) but it is important that there is also consistency of terminology and sharing of information across different professional groups. An example is the discharge summary written from the perspective of one professional group (e.g. the doctor) and not including information from another group also extensively involved with care (e.g. allied health professionals). Lack of physician–nurse record integration of information in a Dallas hospital in 2015 led to a patient with the Ebola virus being sent home inappropriately, and the incident made international news. Trainees in all health professions require education, training and evaluation of their handovers, both verbal and written, to improve patient safety.

The Francis report into the Mid-Staffordshire NHS Foundation Trust identified the ward round as key to good co-ordination of patient care. The nursing team was identified as 'a central point of communication between the patient and medical staff.' Also highlighted in the report were full and comprehensive handovers between shifts, involving members of the multidisciplinary team. Consideration should be given to the timing of ward rounds to maximise participation by all those involved with the patient's care, including the carer and/or the family. Equally, staff should recognise attendance at ward rounds and participation in handovers as being a priority in facilitating clinical communication. Communication within teams is discussed in more detail in Chapter 5.

Written records

The importance of a clear, contemporaneous record is emphasised by professional bodies and accepted as good, safe practice. Deficiencies in written records are related to errors. However, acquisition of this basic skill is not always reflected in training programmes. Review and audit of clinical records are not established elements of appraisal, meaning that suboptimal record-keeping often emerges only when things go wrong. Perhaps more than oral communication, written records are learned through trial and error and are dependent on the role-modelling of senior staff. Similarly, the discharge summary is a crucial piece of communication between the hospital and community services. The quality of discharge summaries is related to clinical workload. Interventions providing teaching and practice of note-keeping and preparation of discharge summaries followed by feedback do improve the abilities of trainees and should be incorporated into core clinical communication training. Defining standards for discharge summaries is also effective. Communication in medical records is discussed in more detail in Chapter 6.

A caring environment

Good clinical communication cannot be commanded or coerced. It is related to an individual's personal characteristics (see Chapter 3) but can also be taught and improved. A stressful, overloaded working environment inhibits effective clinical communication and puts patients at risk. Good organisational management and leadership facilitate good communication, promote job satisfaction and reduce staff turnover. Staff members reporting job satisfaction are more likely to build rapport with patients and display empathy and concern.

Rudeness and incivility can impair clinical performance. Three sources of rudeness have been identified in the healthcare environment:

- hierarchical rudeness – originating from someone in authority;
- peer rudeness – from a colleague;
- client rudeness – enacted by a patient, family member or friend.

All sources of rudeness have the same effect on performance of the recipient. The Francis report also highlighted the attitudes prevalent among staff as contributing to the adverse outcomes for patients found in the hospital. A randomised controlled trial in a simulated neonatal intensive care unit examining the effect of mild rudeness on diagnostic and procedural tasks found that rudeness alone accounted for 12% of the variance between intervention and control groups. This variance increased once information-sharing and help-seeking were accounted for in the analysis. This suggested an effect of incivility on the communication within the intervention team. Composite diagnostic and procedural performance scores were lower for teams exposed to rudeness than for members of control teams.

Conclusions

Communication with patients has always been a key element of the diagnostic process, and it remains so. Good communication underpins the physician–patient relationship (see Box 1.7). An open approach in which patients can describe in detail what is happening to them and what concerns them is important. It is not only a question of determining what is wrong with the patient but also what matters most to the patient. This is facilitated by

Box 1.7 **The physician–patient relationship**

'To attend those who suffer, a physician must possess not only the scientific knowledge and technical abilities, but also an understanding of human nature. The patient is not just a group of symptoms, damaged organs and altered emotions. The patient is a human being, at the same time worried and hopeful, who is searching for relief, help and trust. The importance of an intimate relationship between patient and physician can never be overstated because in most cases an accurate diagnosis, as well as an effective treatment, relies directly on the quality of this relationship.'

Source: From Hellın (2002). Reproduced with permission of Wiley.

listening and learning to see things the patient's way. It is important for healthcare professionals to understand there is an evidence-base for the skills to achieve this and it is important for teachers to define learning objectives to teach these. There remain challenges in making health services truly patient-centred and further research is required to decide which interventions best achieve safe and patient-centred care. Effective information flow within and between healthcare teams is a particular challenge, and training in written communication needs to be given greater priority. Poor communication has a direct effect on patient care. The working environment, including the level of mutual respect and civility, is fundamental to clinical communication between all staff and their patients.

References

Bachmann C, Abramovitch H, Barbu CG. European consensus on learning objectives for a core communication curriculum in health care professions. Pat Educ Couns 2013; 93: 18–26.

Bird J, Cohen-Cole SA. The three function model of the medical interview: an education device. Adv Psychosom Med 1990; 20: 60–88.

Brown J, Noble LM, Papageorgiou A, Kidd J. Clinical Communication in Medicine. Wiley, 2016.

Brown J, Stewart M, McCracken E *et al.* The patient-centred clinical method. 2. Definition and application. Fam Pract 1986; 3: 75–79.

Engel GL. The need for a new medical model: a challenge for biomedicine. Science 1977; 196(4286): 129–36

Fortin AH, Dwamena FC, Frankel RM, Smith RC. Smith's Patient-Centred Interviewing: an Evidence-Based Method, 3rd edn. Columbus, OH: McGraw-Hill Global Education, 2012.

Frankel RM, Stein T. Getting the most out of the clinical encounter: The four habits model. J Med Pract Man 2001; 16: 184–191.

Hellın T. The physician-patient relationship: recent developments and changes. Haemophilia 2002; 8: 450–454.

Kaba R, Sooriakumararan P. The evolution of the doctor-patient relationship. Int J Surg 2007; 5; 57–65.

Keller VF, Carroll JG. A new model for physician-patient communication. Pat Educ Couns 1994; 23:131–140.

Makoul G. Essential elements of communication in medical encounters: The Kalamazoo Consensus Statement. Acad Med 2001; 76: 390–393.

Mead N, Bower P. Patient-centredness: a conceptual framework and review of the empirical literature. Soc Sci Med 2000; 51: 1087–1110.

Platt FM, McMath JC. Clinical hypocompetence: the medical interview. Ann Intern Med 1979; 91(6): 898–902.

Riskin A, Erez A, Foulk TA *et al*. The impact of rudeness on medical team performance: a randomised trial. Pediatrics 2015; 136(3): 487–495.

Silverman JD, Kurtz SM, Draper J. Skills for communicating with patients. Oxford, UK: Radcliffe Medical Press, 1998.

Smith RC, Marshall-Dorsey AA, Osborn GG *et al*. Evidence-based guidelines for patient-centred interviewing. Pat Educ Couns 2000; 39:27–36

Stoeckle JD, Billings AJ. A history of history-taking. J Gen Int Med 1987; 2: 119–127.

Tallman K, Janisse T, Frankel RM *et al*. Communication practices of physicians with high patient-satisfaction ratings. Permanente J 2007; 11(1): 19–29.

Further resources

Beckman HB, Frankel RM. Effect on physician behaviour on the collection of data. Ann Intern Med 1984; 101(5): 692–696.

Francis R. Report of the Mid Staffordshire NHS Foundation Trust Public Enquiry. London: Stationary Office, 2013.

Hampton JR, Harrison MJ, Mitchel JR *et al*. Relative contributions of history-taking, physical examination and laboratory investigations to diagnosis and management of medical outpatients. Br Med J 1975; 2(5969): 486–489.

Riskin A, Erez A, Foulk TA *et al*. The impact of rudeness on medical team performance: a randomised trial. Pediatrics 2015; 136(3): 487–495.

Royal College of Physicians of London and Royal College of Nursing. Ward Rounds in Medicine: Principles for Best Practice. London: RCP, 2012.

CHAPTER 2

The Consultation

Jonathan Silverman

University of Cambridge, Cambridge, UK

OVERVIEW

- The consultation is a highly skilled, complex professional challenge that needs careful attention.
- Extensive research shows that the use of specific communication skills can produce more effective consultations for both doctor and patient.
- The interview can be conceptualised as a set of core tasks, broadly applicable to all healthcare interactions, which can then be further subdivided into a number of discrete, observable behavioural skills.
- The Calgary-Cambridge guide is presented as an example of a conceptual model – then a single real consultation is analysed to demonstrate the importance of effective communication in the accuracy, supportiveness and efficiency of routine consultations.
- To achieve safe, effective, high-quality care, it is important to pay as much attention to the skills of effective communication as to developing excellence in knowledge, practical skills and clinical reasoning.

Introduction

The consultation is central to clinical practice. It is the essential unit of medical time, critical minutes in which the doctor tries to understand the patient and help them with their problems. Whatever else might happen to medical practice in years to come, the face-to-face consultation will undoubtedly remain the key to providing effective high quality healthcare.

It is not easy to get the consultation right: it is a highly skilled, complex, multi-faceted and professional challenge that needs careful attention and cannot be left to chance. It requires thoughtful consideration and planning.

To achieve an effective consultation, doctors need to be able to integrate four aspects of their work which together determine their overall clinical competence (see Box 2.1). These four essential components of clinical competence are inextricably linked. Outstanding

Box 2.1 Four aspects determining clinical competence

- Knowledge
- Communication skills
- Problem-solving
- Physical examination

expertise in any one alone is not sufficient. Communication binds all of this together; if you cannot communicate effectively to obtain an accurate history and make an effective diagnosis, to explore the patient's concerns, to examine the patient sensitively, to explain appropriately and to make collaborative plans, all your knowledge and skills can so easily go to waste.

In the past, the consultation was described only in terms of its output – the information needed from the patient in order to make a diagnosis, or given to a patient in an explanation. This is the *content* of communication. Even less attention was paid to how to build a relationship with the patient or how to organise and structure an interview. Only more recently has attention been paid to how to go about the *process* of information-gathering and -giving, and what communication skills or techniques would aid the retrieval of data required by the doctor and promote the understanding and decision-making of the patient.

There is also a strong argument that the traditional consultation was too restrictive, focusing only on the symptoms and signs of disease that help the clinician to make a diagnosis, at the expense of gathering information about and subsequently addressing the patient's perspective of their illness and, in particular, their ideas, concerns, expectations and feelings.

This chapter looks at the consultation more widely and attempts to integrate all these different elements: content as well as process; the biomedical disease as well as the patient's perspective; clinical reasoning as well as feelings. It will present a model that attempts to incorporate all these elements into a seamless whole, a balanced 'comprehensive clinical method' (see Figure 2.1).

ABC of Clinical Communication, First Edition. Edited by Nicola Cooper and John Frain.
© 2018 John Wiley & Sons Ltd. Published 2018 by John Wiley & Sons Ltd.

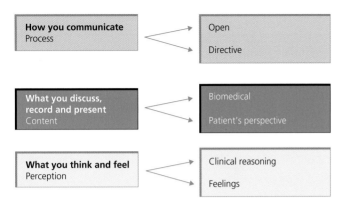

Figure 2.1 A 'comprehensive' clinical method.

Box 2.2 **Effective communication skills and improved clinical performance**

- Good communication is not just about 'being nice' but produces a more effective consultation for both the patient and the doctor.
- Effective communication significantly improves:
  - Accuracy, efficiency and supportiveness
  - Health outcomes for patients
  - Satisfaction for both patient and doctor
  - The therapeutic relationship.
- Communication bridges the gap between evidence-based medicine and working with individual patients.

Evidence-based communication

Perhaps the most important message from the extensive research into the consultation over the last 30 years is that effective communication is not the 'art of medicine', an optional fluffy add-on extra, but part of the science of medicine itself. Indeed, the prize on offer from effective communication skills is improved clinical performance. This is summarised in Box 2.2.

Extensive communication research shows that the use of specific skills can produce more effective consultations for both doctor and patient. Communication skills can make history-taking and problem-solving more accurate and help us to be more supportive to patients. The appropriate use of communication skills enables us to be more efficient in day-to-day practice in the real world. Indeed, research correlates the use of individual skills with improvements in all the following parameters of care: patient satisfaction, adherence, symptom relief and physiological outcome.

Communication can also improve outcomes for doctors. The use of appropriate communication skills can not only increase patient satisfaction with their doctors but also help doctors to feel less frustrated and more satisfied in their work. Not least, effective communication reduces patient complaints.

In this chapter, we discuss communication approaches that support a patient-centred methodology and promote a collaborative partnership between patient and health professional. This is not a matter of subjective opinion or personal belief – the skills that operationalise this theoretical approach to the doctor–patient relationship have been shown, in both research and practice, to produce better outcomes for patients and doctors.

The concept of a collaborative partnership implies a more equal relationship between patient and doctor, and a shift in the balance of power away from medical paternalism towards mutuality. This chapter enumerates the communication skills that doctors can employ to enhance their patients' ability to become more involved in the consultation and to take part in a more balanced relationship.

Models of the consultation

The importance of structure

Practitioners, learners and teachers of healthcare communication all require a means of conceptualising the complex process of the consultation, of organising what is inherently a highly dynamic process into manageable elements. Without some form of structural model, it is all too easy for consultations to be unsystematic or unproductive and for experiential communication teaching to appear random and opportunistic. Paradoxically, structure sets us free – it provides us with an awareness of the distinct phases of the interview as we consult and the flexibility to move away from a fixed path when appropriate, with the security of understanding how to return to our structure in due course.

Core tasks, core skills and specific issues

In order to provide this degree of organisation, the healthcare interview can be conceptualised as a set of core tasks, broadly applicable to all healthcare interactions. These tasks can then be further subdivided into a number of discrete, observable, specific behavioural skills relevant to the execution of each task. These core tasks and skills provide the foundations for effective practitioner-patient communication in a variety of different clinical contexts, providing a secure platform for approaching many specific communication issues.

Core tasks and skills are of fundamental importance: once they have been mastered, specific communication challenges such as anger, addiction, breaking bad news or diversity issues are much more readily tackled. This platform of core tasks and skills serves as the primary resource for dealing with all challenges. Rather than inventing a new set of skills for each issue, we need to consider how to use particular subsets of skills with greater intention, intensity and awareness. This interrelationship between tasks, skills and issues is well represented in the curriculum wheel developed by the UK Council of Clinical Communication in Undergraduate Medical Education (see 'Further resources') and illustrated in Figure 2.2.

A number of widely used consultation models and frameworks have been developed by teachers and researchers which list these skills and tasks in a variety of ways (see 'Further resources'). Here we describe the Calgary-Cambridge guide, our own conceptual model.

The Calgary-Cambridge guide

The Calgary-Cambridge guide uses the following structure of seven tasks – five sequential tasks which represent the natural flow of the consultation and would be instantly recognisable to any clinician, and two continuous threads (building the relationship and providing structure) which require constant attention

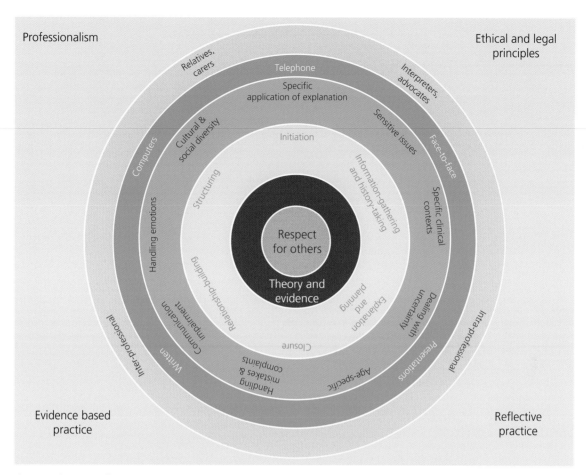

Figure 2.2 The curriculum wheel for clinical communication. *Source*: Von Fragstein *et al*. (2008). Reproduced with permission of the UK Council of Clinical Communication in Undergraduate Medical Education.

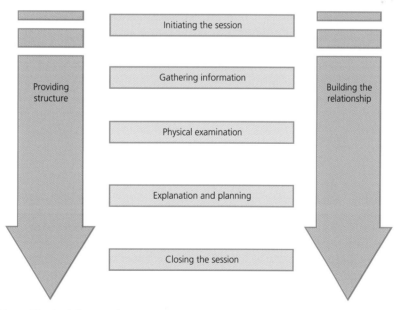

Figure 2.3 The Calgary-Cambridge guide – basic framework.

throughout the consultation in order to enable the sequential tasks to be achieved effectively (see Figure 2.3)

These tasks can then be subdivided by identifying the objectives to be achieved within each communication task (see Figure 2.4).

In the Calgary-Cambridge guide, the framework provides an overview that helps the learner or practitioner to organise and apply the behaviourally specific, evidence-based communication process skills which are then listed under each objective (see Figure 2.5).

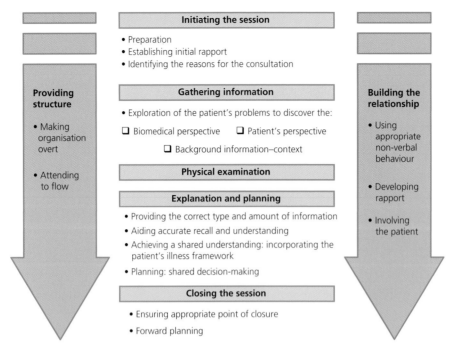

Figure 2.4 The Calgary-Cambridge Guide – the expanded framework.

An example of the importance of the model in practice

Rather than try to explore any of these specific skills in detail, I would like to give an example of a recent consultation witnessed by myself when I accompanied a patient to a review appointment in a cardiology clinic in a centre of excellence in the UK.

A fit and well 92-year-old woman had recently had a coronary artery stent for angina at rest despite maximal anti-anginal therapy. In the 4 weeks since the procedure, she had been able to return to walking to the shops on a daily basis without any pain. However, the week before, she had had an episode of severe chest pain and had been admitted to another hospital in the locality. She had been discharged with the advice that it probably was not her heart but either musculoskeletal or indigestion pain.

In the clinic, she was seen by a Registrar (Intern), whom she had not met before, who was kindly, knowledgeable, intelligent and clearly very competent. It is interesting how much confidence can be built in such a very short time at the beginning of a consultation. He *greeted* her warmly by her name, gave effective *eye contact*, *introduced* himself and his role and was very *respectful*. He was disadvantaged by the layout of the room in which the patient was at the opposite side of a large desk and he had to turn away from her to look at the computer screen, which she could not see at all.

So he had *established initial rapport* effectively according to the Calgary-Cambridge skills. However, it was in the *identification of the reasons for the consultation* that things became less effective. He recapped what had happened to the patient before she was discharged while running through the information on the screen. But he used a lot of *technical language* which the patient did not understand and missed the opportunity of *picking up her cues* because he did not make *eye contact* at this stage. He then asked her two very

specific *closed questions*: 'Have you had any further pain when out walking to the shops?,' and 'Have you had any pain at night?,' to which she correctly answered, 'No'. He did not ask any *open questions* such as 'How have you been since your procedure?' and did not *screen* for any problems she wanted to discuss today or *set an agenda* for the meeting.

There was little *attentive listening* or *facilitation*. He did not discover the patient's *concerns* and worries and therefore was not able to *empathise* with them. A combination of lack of attention to *non-verbal behaviour* and *rapport building* at this stage meant that she became more passive in the consultation and despite a natural tendency to be talkative, she became quiet. He also did not use the twin skills of *summarising* and *signposting* to structure the consultation and so the patient got somewhat lost in the consultation and did not know when it was appropriate to speak.

The Registrar then moved to *explanation and planning* and rather than use *chunking and checking* or *assessing the starting point* of the patient, he gave a lot of information in one go with a very large number of *jargon* words which the patient did not understand. However, he was very upbeat, explained the procedure had been a very great success and that he was very pleased with her progress and they should meet again in 1 year's time. He did not ask if she had any *questions or concerns* about what he had said or *check her understanding*. But he was very charming and kindly.

The problem with this consultation is that the patient would have left at this point and the following issues would have been left unattended:

1   The doctor, despite his best intentions, would not have found out the highly important history of the recurrence of chest pain following the procedure and the subsequent admission to hospital and therefore he employed inappropriate clinical reasoning and decision-making.

INITIATING THE SESSION

Establish initial rapport
Greet patient and obtains patient's name
Introduce self, role and nature of interview; obtain consent
Demonstrate respect and interest, attend to patient's physical comfort

Identify the reason(s) for the consultation
Use appropriate **opening question** to identify problems/issues
Listen attentively to opening statement without interruption
Confirm list and **screen** for further problems
Negotiate agenda

GATHERING INFORMATION

Explore patient's problems
Encourage patient to **tell the story** from when first started
Use **open to closed cone**
Listen attentively
Facilitate patient's responses verbally and non-verbally
Pick up verbal and non-verbal **cues**
Clarify statements
Periodically **summarise**
Use concise, easily understood **language**
Establish **dates**

Understand the patient's perspective
Determine, acknowledge and appropriately explore:
• patient's **ideas** and **concerns**
• patient's **expectations**
• how each problem **affects** the patient's life
Encourage expression of the patient's **feelings**

BUILDING THE RELATIONSHIP

Use appropriate non-verbal behaviour
Demonstrate appropriate **non–verbal behaviour:**
• eye contact, facial expression
• posture, position and movement
• vocal cues, e.g. rate, volume, tone
If writing **notes,** ensure does not interfere with dialogue or rapport

Develop rapport
Accept patient's views and feelings non-judgmentally
Use **empathy**, acknowledge feelings and predicament
Provide **support**
Deal **sensitively** with embarrassing and disturbing topics, pain

Involve the patient
Share thinking with patient
Explain rationale for questions
During **physical examination**, explain process/ask permission

PROVIDING STRUCTURE TO THE CONSULTATION

Make organisation overt
Summarise at the end of a specific line of inquiry
Signpost next section

Attend to flow
Structure interview in **logical sequence**
Attend to **timing**

PROVIDING THE CORRECT AMOUNT AND TYPE OF INFORMATION

Chunk and check: give information in manageable chunks, use patient's response as guide to how to proceed
Assess patient's starting point: ask for patient's prior knowledge, discover extent of patient's wish for information
Discover what other information would help patient
e.g. aetiology, prognosis
Give explanation at appropriate times: avoid giving advice, information or reassurance prematurely

AIDING ACCURATE RECALL AND UNDERSTANDING

Organise explanation: divide into discrete sections, develop a logical sequence
Use explicit categorisation or signposting (e.g. 'There are three important things that I would like to discuss. First...' 'Now, shall we move on to.')
Use repetition and summarising to reinforce information
Use concise, easily understood language, avoid or explain jargon
Use visual methods of conveying information: diagrams, models, written information and instructions
Check patient's understanding of information given, e.g. by asking patient to restate in own words; clarify as necessary

ACHIEVING A SHARED UNDERSTANDING: INCORPORATING THE PATIENT'S PERSPECTIVE

Relate explanations to patient's illness framework: to previously elicited ideas, concerns and expectations
Provide opportunities and encourage patient to contribute: to ask questions, seek clarification or express doubts; respond appropriately
Pick up non-verbal and covert verbal cues, e.g. patient's need to contribute information or ask questions, information overload, distress
Elicit patient's beliefs, reactions and feelings re: information given, terms used, acknowledge and address where necessary

PLANNING: SHARED DECISION-MAKING

Share own thinking as appropriate: ideas, thought processes, dilemmas
Involve patient:
• offer suggestions and choices rather than directives
• encourage patient to contribute their own ideas, suggestions
Explore management options
Ascertain level of involvement patient wishes in making the decision at hand
Negotiate a mutually acceptable plan:
• signpost own position of equipoise or preference regarding available options
• determine patient's preferences
Check with patient:
• if accepts plans
• if concerns have been addressed

CLOSING THE SESSION

Forward planning
Contract with patient re. next steps for patient and physician
Safety net, explaining possible unexpected outcomes, what to do if plan is not working, when and how to seek help

Ensuring appropriate point of closure
Summarise session briefly and clarify plan of care
Final check that patient agrees and is comfortable with plan and ask if any corrections, questions or other items to discuss

Figure 2.5 The Calgary-Cambridge Guide – communication process skills.

2 The patient's concerns had not been addressed:

   a She had been upset at being readmitted to hospital. Following the procedure, she was told that if she had any further chest pain this would definitely not be from her heart and so she delayed calling for help despite severe pain, and yet on admission to another hospital, they took the possibility of the pain coming from the heart very seriously and implied she should have come earlier.

   b She wanted to know what to do if the pain occurred again and what the cause was. If it was indigestion, should she stop taking aspirin?

3 The information given to the patient was inappropriate.

4 The patient did not understand the information that she was given.

What is so interesting here is that the patient and I had rehearsed exactly what she wanted to say in the waiting room before she went in and it was on the tip of her tongue. She knew she wanted to ask about her admission to hospital, as she realised that the doctor might not know about it, and she wanted to explain her concerns and have her questions answered. But the format of the interview strongly prevented her from doing this. She was also impressed by the young man and felt he was competent and knowledgeable and would not have known at this point in the consultation that things had gone awry.

I intervened just before the consultation ended and asked the patient if she had managed to say all the things she wanted to. As a result, the poor doctor had to retrace all his steps and start again, having discovered a new history which influenced his decision-making, explanation and follow-up plans. I felt sorry for him, not just because I could have intervened earlier, but also because he was so well-intentioned, trying to be both helpful and careful but let down by not using the appropriate set of skills to run a review consultation, which I suspect he had never been taught. In essence, the consultation lacked accuracy in history-taking and became inefficient because of the need to redo much of what had happened. By not addressing the woman's concerns, it was unsupportive, even if the patient did not really appreciate this.

Conclusions

The consultation is a complex task, which brings all of the skills of medicine together in one brief episode. In the past, doctors have paid considerable attention to only certain elements of this. Teachers have always been quite adamant that excellence in knowledge, clinical skills and clinical reasoning were the hallmarks of high-quality healthcare. In this chapter, we have demonstrated the key role of communication alongside and fully integrated with these other components, and shown the importance of paying as much attention to learning the process skills of effective communication in the consultation in order to achieve safe, effective, high-quality care.

Acknowledgements

I would like to acknowledge my co-authors in our previous books and papers, Suzanne Kurtz, Juliet Draper and John Benson, for help with the development of the concepts presented here.

Reference

Von Fragstein M, Silverman J, Cushing A *et al*. UK consensus statement on the content of communication curricula in undergraduate medical education. Med Educ 2008; 42 (11): 1100–1107.

Further resources

European Association for Communication in Healthcare (EACH). www.each.eu (Accessed January 2017).

Kurtz S, Silverman J, Benson J, Draper J. Marrying content and process in clinical method teaching: Enhancing the Calgary-Cambridge Guides. Acad Med 2003; 78(8): 802–809.

Silverman J. Teaching clinical communication: a mainstream activity or just a minority sport? Patient Educ Counsel 2009; 76(3): 361–367.

Silverman J, Kurtz SM, Draper J. Skills for Communicating with Patients, 3rd edn. Oxford, UK: Radcliffe, 2013.

Stewart MA, Brown JB, Weston WW *et al*. Patient-Centered Medicine: Transforming the Clinical Method, 3rd edn. Oxford, UK: Radcliffe Medical Press, 2013.

CHAPTER 3

Communication and Personality Type

Gillian B. Clack

King's College London, London, UK

> **OVERVIEW**
>
> - Diverse factors affect communication between individuals.
> - Personality type differences are one powerful factor.
> - Jung's theory of personality type differences is described here.
> - How these relate to the consultation process is explained.
> - Healthcare professionals can learn to 'flex' their communication style to match their patients.

Introduction

You have read in previous chapters the importance of good communication in achieving patient satisfaction and compliance. Different models of consultation have been described, including the importance of listening skills and the contexts in which these are particularly important, such as breaking bad news, difficult consultations and in the field of mental health.

As individuals we tend to see the world through our own individual lenses, and communication can therefore be affected by such factors as our culture, gender, class, education, upbringing, religion, and so on. So clinicians need to be mindful of these in their interactions (and potential clashes) with their patients and other team members.

One other powerful difference that is relevant concerns the personality types of those involved in the interaction. We have all experienced situations in which we tune in immediately to the person with whom we are in conversation, whereas, in other cases, we just do not seem to be on the same wavelength and it is a bit of a struggle. This is often due to our personality type differences, so one size does not fit all in a consultation situation. It is important to understand, therefore, what information patients with different personality types want and to use language that is clear and meaningful to them.

This chapter will explore the theory behind personality type and then go on to describe how these differences may affect communication between healthcare professionals and their patients and how 'flexing' one's consultation style can move towards a more satisfactory interaction and outcome.

Jung's theory of personality type

In order for effective communication to occur between two individuals there needs to be a 'meeting of minds'. Personality type, or psychological type to be more correct, as measured by the Myers–Briggs Type Indicator (MBTI) can help to demonstrate similarities and differences in how people process the kind of material doctors and patients regularly discuss. It has been shown that couples with a similar communication style, or those who can easily adjust to the communication style preferences of others, derive more satisfaction from the resulting relationship.

The Swiss psychiatrist Carl Jung observed that when one's mind is active it is involved in one of two mental processes: taking in information, which he called 'perceiving' or organising that information, and coming to conclusions about it, which he called 'judging'. He found that there were two opposite ways of 'perceiving', which he called 'sensing' and 'intuition', and two opposite ways of 'judging' which he called 'thinking' and 'feeling'. However, everyone uses all four processes every day in the outer world of things and people ('extraversion') and the inner world of ideas and reflections ('introversion'). Jung believed, however, that individuals have preferences between these opposites, which are inborn or 'hard-wired' and explain why some processes come more easily and naturally to us, whereas others require more concentration and effort, e.g. like being right- or left-handed.

The theory was further developed by Briggs and Myers who incorporated, in addition, the way individuals like to live their lives and orientate themselves to the outside world, i.e. primarily using their 'judging' or 'perceiving' process. These four bipolar dichotomies are the building blocks that make up personality type (see Figure 3.1).

Myers went on to develop a psychometric instrument, the MBTI, to help Jung's theory become accessible to individuals by identifying their preferred ways of mental processing along these dichotomies, resulting in the 16 personality types that are now familiar to many of us. It has been shown to be a valid and reliable instrument and is one of the most widely used personality questionnaires in the world.

ABC of Clinical Communication, First Edition. Edited by Nicola Cooper and John Frain.
© 2018 John Wiley & Sons Ltd. Published 2018 by John Wiley & Sons Ltd.

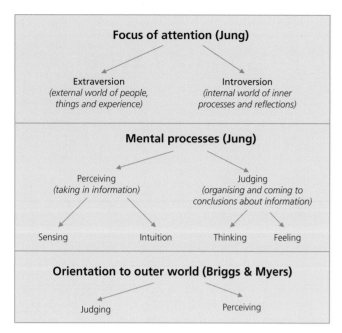

Figure 3.1 Jung's theory of psychological type. *Source:* Clack *et al.* (2004). Reproduced with permission of Wiley.

Box 3.1 **Focus of attention: extraversion versus introversion**

Extraversion	Introversion
• Are very aware of the external environment	• Are drawn to their own internal world
• Like to communicate by talking – processing out loud	• Like to communicate in writing – processing internally
• Learn best through action and discussion	• Learn best by reflecting and mental practice
• Have a wide breadth of interests	• Have a depth of interest
• Have a tendency to speak first and reflect later	• Tend to reflect before acting or speaking
• Are sociable, dynamic and expressive	• Are private people, self-contained
• Take the initiative in work and relationships	• Find focusing easy

---

Extraverted versus introverted attitude

The MBTI identifies firstly where individuals prefer to focus their attention, where they get their energy and buzz, in either the outer world of things and people (extraversion) or the inner world of ideas and experiences (introversion).

Those who prefer extraversion usually like to communicate by talking, learn best through actively doing something, develop their ideas by discussing them, and tend to speak first and reflect later.

People who prefer introversion, however, generally like to communicate by writing, work out ideas and learn best by reflection and mental practice, and prefer time to think before acting or speaking (see Box 3.1).

Sensing versus intuitive perception

Secondly, the instrument reveals how people prefer to take in information and learn about things, either through their five senses with a focus on the present (sensing perception) or by seeing the 'big picture' with a focus on the future (intuitive perception).

Individuals preferring sensing perception like to take in information through their five senses – to find out what is happening in the present, what is real and tangible. They are very observant, take note of detail and are particularly attuned to practical realities. They prefer to deal in facts, what is concrete and grounded, before moving on to the abstract, taking in information step by step, starting from what is familiar, as they observe and remember sequentially. They value practical applications as illustrations in order to understand theory.

In contrast, those who prefer intuitive perception like to take in information by seeing the 'big picture' rather than the details, looking ahead for possibilities and opportunities in the future, and seeking relationships and connections between facts. Their attention is drawn to things that stimulate their imagination, their minds working in skips and jumps, looking for patterns and new insights wherever the inspiration takes them. They like to clarify ideas and theories before putting them into practice (see Box 3.2).

Thinking versus feeling judgment

Thirdly, the MBTI identifies how individuals like to process and come to conclusions about the information they have received. Those who prefer the thinking mode of decision-making tend to step back mentally from a situation and examine it dispassionately, analysing the pros and cons and logical consequences of a choice or course of action, aimed at an impersonal finding that is consistent with the objective data. They have a strong belief in justice and fairness, wanting everyone treated equally.

On the other hand, those who prefer the feeling mode of decision-making tend to concentrate on what is important to them and other people affected. They decide, with reference to their

---

Box 3.2 **How people prefer to take in information: sensing versus intuitive perception**

Sensing	Intuitive
• Focus on what is real, actual and grounded	• Focus on 'big picture', new possibilities and opportunities
• Prefer to see practical applications	• Value imaginative insight
• Are factual, concrete and realistic	• Tend to be abstract and theoretical
• Are aware of and easily remember details	• Look for and see patterns and meanings in facts
• Tend to observe and remember sequentially	• Look to the future
• Have a focus on the past and present	• Minds jump around from one thing to another
• Like to receive information step by step	• Trust inspiration
• Trust experience and what has worked before	

Box 3.3 **How people make decisions: thinking versus feeling judgment**

Thinking	Feeling
• Focus on logical analysis in decision-making	• Focus on person-centred values in decision-making – what is the 'right' thing to do
• Seek to be impersonal and objective	• Assess impact of decisions on people
• Use cause-and-effect reasoning	• Are sympathetic and compassionate
• Enjoy problem-solving	• Tend to be 'tender-hearted' – may avoid tough decisions
• Can take the tough decisions if necessary	• Strive for harmony
• Strive to be reasonable and fair	

Box 3.4 **How people deal with the outer world: judging or perceiving orientation**

Judging	Perceiving
• Like things organised and under control	• Flexible and adaptable
• Tend to draw up plans and schedules	• Spontaneous – plans can be constraining if there is no room for adaptation
• Prefer systematic and methodical approach to life	• Tend to adopt a 'go with the flow' approach to life
• Get great satisfaction from completing tasks or deciding things	• Like to stay open to consider further options before deciding
• Avoid last-minute stresses	• Are energised by last-minute pressures

values, to determine what they believe is the right thing to do. They mentally place themselves in a situation and identify with the people involved so their decisions can take account of the effect on themselves and others and their ideal outcome is harmony. They too want fairness but they want everyone treated as an individual.

Those learning about personality type theory often confuse these terms and imagine that 'thinking' is logical and uncaring and 'feeling' is emotional and irrational. The very terms Jung chose can, indeed, add to this confusion. However, he was quite clear that both thinking and feeling judgement are rational ways of making decisions – they just focus on different criteria (see Box 3.3).

Judging versus perceiving orientation

The fourth dichotomy, identified later by Briggs and Myers, is how individuals like to live their lives and orientate themselves to the outer world. Briggs had observed that there were different behavioural characteristics associated with those who lead with their perceiving function (sensing or intuition) and those who lead with their judging function (thinking or feeling).

Those who use their judging process in the outside world exhibit decisiveness, a willingness to apply themselves to tasks, like system and order in the present and long-range plans in the future. They tend, therefore, to live in a planned, orderly way, wanting to have their lives under control. They like to have things settled, and sticking to a plan and schedule is important to them. They get great satisfaction from completing tasks and dislike last-minute stresses.

In contrast, those who use their perceiving function in the outside world usually show curiosity, receptiveness, spontaneity and adaptability to change. They tend to live in a more flexible, spontaneous way, seeking to experience life rather than control it. Detailed plans and decisions feel confining to them if there is no scope for adaptation, and they prefer to stay open to experience and last-minute options. They trust and enjoy their resourcefulness and adaptability to respond to the demands of the situation (see Box 3.4).

However, it is important to remember that we all use every one of these mental processes every day of our lives depending upon context. It is just that some come more naturally to us and we tend to go there first. This has been likened to inhabiting a house where we may go from room to room during the day as appropriate but there

is always one room where we feel most at home, and this is what type is like. So, one's personality type preference is not putting you in a box – it just illustrates what is likely to come most easily to you, your default position.

Jung's theory of psychological type has recently found strong support in the scientific research of Professor Nardi at the University of California, Los Angeles. Using electroencephalogram (EEG) neuro-mapping equipment, he studied the neocortical activity of people with the various personality types as they engaged in a variety of tasks for several hours. He found that the brain activity exhibited did, indeed, relate to Jung's eight cognitive processes, each type using their brains in fundamentally different ways. So neuroscience now supports what Jung found in his case studies nearly 100 years ago.

Are doctors' preferences different?

Having read the descriptions of the different personality types, you may have developed some idea of your own type preferences and feel it would be useful to explore this newly acquired self-awareness further. If so, it is recommended that this is done with the aid of a qualified MBTI practitioner as there are many instruments on the internet purporting to identify personality type, but most are not validated and so should be treated with caution.

In research conducted by the author of this chapter, as far as the preferred mode of perception was concerned (sensing/intuition), the difference between doctors and the UK population was marked, with under half preferring sensing compared with over three-quarters of the UK population. There were also fewer doctors with the combination of sensing with thinking (ST), significantly fewer with sensing with feeling (SF), but significantly more with intuition with feeling (NF) and intuition with thinking (NT) than in the UK population (see Figure 3.2). Consequently, a patient with a preference for sensing with feeling (40.1% of the UK population) would have only a 1 in 6 chance of seeing a doctor with the same preferences. Similarly, a doctor with preferences for intuition and thinking (31.3% of this sample) would have only a 1 in 11 chance that the patient was similar to them.

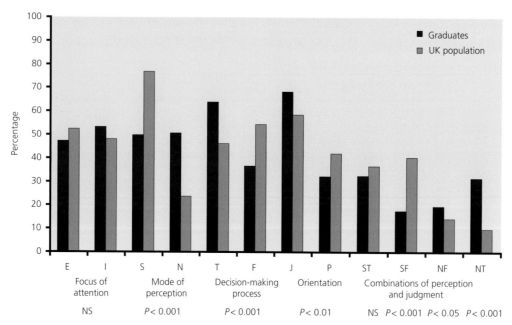

Figure 3.2 Personality preferences of medical graduates ($n=313$) compared with UK adults ($n=1634$). E, extraversion; I, introversion; S, sensing perception; N, intuitive perception; T, thinking judgment; F, feeling judgment; J, judging orientation; P, perceiving orientation; ST, sensing perception with thinking judgment; SF, sensing perception with feeling judgment; NF, intuitive perception with feeling judgment; NT, intuitive perception with thinking judgment. *Source:* Clack *et al.* (2004). Reproduced with permission of Wiley.

Thus, it is easy to see that once you are aware of your own preferences, finding ways of adapting to those who are different could enhance your clinical practice.

How type differences relate to communication

As individuals we tend to communicate with others in the way we ourselves prefer to receive communication, but this does not always work if the other party has different type preferences. It is not, however, necessary for you to know the personality type of your patient in the consultation, as they may not exhibit the usual cues for their true type. People tend to use different aspects of type at different times depending on context. What you need to identify, therefore, is the 'type mode' they are showing at the time they meet you, as this will affect what they look for in the consultation.

Clues to this can be found in different behavioural cues shown during the consultation, which you can learn to pick up. You can then 'flex' your consultation style to meet what the patient is looking for in that particular healthcare situation by using appropriate language. As individuals mature, however, it is likely they will have more fully developed their type preferences, so experienced clinicians will probably instinctively pick up on these cues and 'flex' their consultation style accordingly, but what follows is a framework that can assist with this process.

This draws on the work of Allen and Brock, based on their research with a large number of patients and healthcare practitioners in order to identify what people found important when receiving healthcare. What they discovered was that the most powerful predictor of how a person prefers to be communicated with in this context was, indeed, consistent with the respondents' type preferences. They then developed a framework to assist healthcare

practitioners tune in to the needs of their patients, using these type preferences and how they were exhibited.

They proposed a four-part framework to describe the consultation process, starting with the first encounter with the patient, (1) 'initiating the interaction', followed by (2) a process of 'investigating needs', moving on to (3) 'suggesting a course of action' and, finally, (4) the 'next steps or closing'.

Thus, in the first encounter, whether a patient exhibits characteristics of extraversion or introversion may be observed. Then during (2) and (3), when the heart of the problem is discussed, the preferred mode of taking in information (sensing or intuitive perception) and decision-making (thinking or feeling judgment) will be at the forefront. Finally, at the end of the consultation (4), whether the patient likes closure or a more open approach (judging or perceiving orientation) will be relevant.

Box 3.5 shows the characteristics of the Myers–Briggs Type Indicator (MBTI) personality preferences as expressed in the context of communication.

Having identified your patient's likely 'type mode' the aim will be to communicate with him/her in a way that will place you both on the same wavelength. Allen and Brock found that this worked best when the functional pairs : sensing with thinking (ST), sensing with feeling (SF), intuition with thinking (NT) and intuition with feeling (NF) were used as outlined in Box 3.6, illustrated with some quotes from patients.

When it comes to 'next steps' or 'closing', healthcare professionals reported that patients who preferred the judging orientation described the importance of providing some structure to the situation and getting an end result, whereas those with the perceiving orientation tended to relate to the process of working together, not the outcome (see Box 3.7). In summary, the STs have a focus on the facts, well-ordered and delivered with the minimum of fuss.

Box 3.5 Characteristics of the Myers–Briggs Type Indicator (MBTI) personality preferences as expressed in the context of communication

PREFERRED FOCUS OF ATTENTION

Extraversion
- Appears to think aloud
- Interrupts
- Louder volume of voice

Introversion
- Pauses while giving information
- Shorter sentences – not run on
- Quieter voice volume

PREFERRED MODE OF TAKING IN INFORMATION

Sensing
- Asks for step by step information or instruction
- Asks 'What?' and 'How?' questions
- Uses precise descriptions

Intuition
- Asks for current and long-term implications
- Asks 'Why?' questions
- Talks in general terms

PREFERRED BASIS FOR DECISION MAKING

Thinking
- Appears to be testing you or your knowledge
- Weighs the objective evidence
- Not impressed that others have decided in favour

Feeling
- Strives for harmony in interaction
- May talk about what they value
- Asks how others acted/resolved the situation

PREFERRED APPROACH TO MANAGING ONE'S LIFE

Judging
- Impatient with overly long descriptions or procedures
- The tone is 'Let's get it done'
- May even decide prematurely and not want to listen to important considerations

Perceiving
- Conversation may move through many areas
- May feel put off by closing a conversation before they're ready
- No decision before its time – often at last minute or when absolutely necessary in their view

Source: Allen and Brock (2002). Reproduced with permission.

Box 3.6 Communication styles preferred by individuals with different Myers–Briggs Type Indicator (MBTI) preferences

FACTS WITH PRACTICALITY
(*'sensing' perception with 'thinking' judgment*)
- Be brief, give concise facts
- Be straightforward and honest
- Know the facts about my condition and expect to be questioned on them
- Present the information in a logical way, do not go off on a tangent

'I just want the straightforward facts, no fuzzy prelude.' ('sensing with thinking' patient)

PERSONAL SERVICE
(*'sensing' perception with 'feeling' judgment*)
- Listen carefully to me, give me your time and complete attention
- Be warm and friendly
- Give me factual information honestly, but with a personal touch - for example, remember what I've already told you
- Provide practical information and examples about my condition

'I need clear information delivered by someone who relates to me as a person.' ('sensing with feeling' patient)

LOGICAL OPTIONS WITH COMPETENCE
(*'intuitive' perception with 'thinking' judgment*)
- Respect my intelligence and my need to understand
- Demonstrate your competence
- Answer my questions in an honest, open way – do not hide anything
- Give me overall options so I can see a pattern

'I want to know that the doctor is competent, what options there are and to be consulted as an equal.' ('intuitive with thinking' patient)

SUPPORTING THE VISION
(*'intuitive' perception with 'feeling' judgment*)
- Treat me with respect, as a whole person, not a case number
- Listen to and value my concerns
- Provide overall solutions, an overview without details
- Take time to discuss my concerns, be honest but kind

'I want to be seen as a whole person, not a disease, and to have my personal values taken into account.' ('intuitive with feeling' patient)

Source: Allen and Brock (2002). Reproduced with permission.

Box 3.7 Communication styles preferred by individuals with different Myers–Briggs Type Indicator (MBTI) preferences in the context of closing the consultation

Judging types

- Clarify the patient's goals, and when they should be reached for optimal outcome
- Ensure patient does not make decisions on next steps prematurely due to anxiety of waiting
- Have a timetable and stick to it or say why/when a strict schedule may not be observed (e.g. surgery on x date/time unless an emergency shifts the time)
- Expect a push to 'get it done' as soon as possible; offer any tests as soon as possible
- Leave no loose ends; clarify details so that nothing is overlooked in the decision

Perceiving types

- Clarify the patient's goals; give the overall time frame when they should be reached for optimal outcome
- Present all options for action to patient before making decisions on next steps
- Make next steps fit the patient's timetable if possible (e.g. surgery after a birthday)
- Expect a last-minute rush to completion of tests or adherence to deadlines – schedule accordingly
- If possible, allow the decision-making process to stay open until the last minute in case new information is discovered

Source: Adapted by Judith O'Rourke, Leadership Coach, JLO Leadership Coaching & Consulting, LLC, from Allen and Brock (2002).

The priority of NFs is to be seen as individuals with complex personal needs. SFs place the highest value on a caring and personal service, while the NTs seek recognition of their intelligence and demonstration of competence by the professional with whom they are working.

This framework has multiple applications and more can be found in Allen and Brock's work, including breaking bad news, encouraging patients to follow clinical advice, working together within the healthcare team and one's own personal and professional development.

However, the overriding word used by all types in relation to good communication is *listen* – and if we listen closely for the behavioural cues and then respond using a matching 'dialect', the patient will know that we *listened and heard* and be more likely to comply with any proposed treatment plan.

Acknowledgement

I would like to express my thanks to Judy Allen, MA, RGN, co-author of 'Health care communication using personality type: patients are different!' for allowing me to freely use her material in this chapter and for providing valuable insight into the important application of personality type in the healthcare setting.

References

Allen J, Brock SA. FLEX Care® Participant Materials, Gainesville, FL: Center for Application of Psychological Type, 2002.

Clack GB, Allen J, Cooper DJ, Head JO. Personality differences between doctors and their patients: implications for the teaching of communication skills. Med Educ 2004: 38: 177–186.

Further resources

Allen J, Brock SA. Health care communication using personality type: patients are different! London, UK: Routledge, 2000.

Myers IB. Introduction to Type, 6th edn. (European English edition). Oxford, UK: Oxford Psychologists Press, 2000.

Myers IB, Myers PB. Gifts Differing: Understanding Personality Type. Palo Alto, CA: Consultant Psychologists Press, 1993.

Nardi D. Neuroscience of Personality. Los Angeles, CA: Radiance House: 2011. Also online: http://www.radiancehouse.com/itemLG_500.htm. Accessed May 2017.

CHAPTER 4

Shared Decision-Making

John Frain[1] and Andy Wearn[2]

[1] University of Nottingham, Nottingham, UK
[2] University of Auckland, Auckland, New Zealand

OVERVIEW

- Shared decision-making requires a two-way exchange of information between patient and doctor.
- Health-related and personal information may be brought to the discussion by any party (patient, doctor, other professionals or third parties).
- Parties should have an awareness of the evidence base for the condition, treatment or management plan under discussion; depth will vary.
- The doctor's perspective should include an appreciation of the patient's past, present and future experience of the health condition.
- The patient requires an understanding of the risks, benefits and uncertainty of the condition under discussion.

Introduction

In western healthcare systems, patients are often dissatisfied with the extent to which they are involved with decisions affecting their care. Information received by patients may not reflect their need for information. Reported reasons for this include the use of terms and/or language that are too difficult for patients to understand, insufficient information or omissions. In particular, health professionals may not sufficiently check patients' understanding of the issues or their consequences. Techniques enabling professionals to facilitate high-quality shared decision-making with patients may be unknown to the healthcare professional or remain unused.

The burgeoning mountain of accessible health information provides a daunting challenge for health professionals to keep themselves adequately informed and up-to-date, not least from a proliferation of professional guidelines and protocols, but also from sources of varying reliability such as the Internet. Most of the time, healthcare professionals need to inform patients about what is happening to them and what management is proposed. This is so that patients can be as fully informed as possible in order to have freedom of choice about what is happening to them. It should also be remembered that patients are able to access healthcare information and this will influence their starting position, for better or worse.

In terms of impact, studies of the outcomes of shared decision-making show some positive effects for affective and cognitive factors (e.g. feeling less anxious, becoming informed), but the evidence on behaviour change and clinical outcomes is less clear (Shay & Lafata, 2014). This chapter focuses on setting up an environment in which patients are heard, their concerns are addressed and their information needs are met with high-quality evidence.

What do patients want?

Most patients want to be provided with more information about their care. This reflects wider trends in society and across the world of individuals wishing to take more control of their lives, to exercise greater freedom and to be more proactive as 'consumers'. However, there are social and cultural nuances to be considered, e.g. age, individual versus collectivist, hierarchical versus flat. Over the last 30 years, the proportion of patients wishing to participate in decisions about their healthcare has risen to three-quarters. A mismatch between preferred level of participation in decision-making and actual experience induces patient anxiety. Patients tend to make more conservative decisions regarding their health than do their healthcare professionals. The facilitators and barriers to shared decision-making, as perceived by patients, are displayed in Figure 4.1.

What is shared decision-making?

Clearly, there are situations in healthcare when shared decision-making is not a priority, such as in the resuscitation room of an Emergency Department when urgent action is required to save someone's life. But in routine healthcare, patients make decisions about their care and this requires the integration of the best available evidence with the patients' own preferences. This will include their values, beliefs and priorities. This is the essence of 'patient-centredness'. Shared decision-making should enable both patient and doctor to state their understanding and preferences, and to come to a decision together about how best to proceed. It has been suggested that there is a perception mismatch between clinicians thinking that they are patient-centred and genuinely applying that

---

ABC of Clinical Communication, First Edition. Edited by Nicola Cooper and John Frain.
© 2018 John Wiley & Sons Ltd. Published 2018 by John Wiley & Sons Ltd.

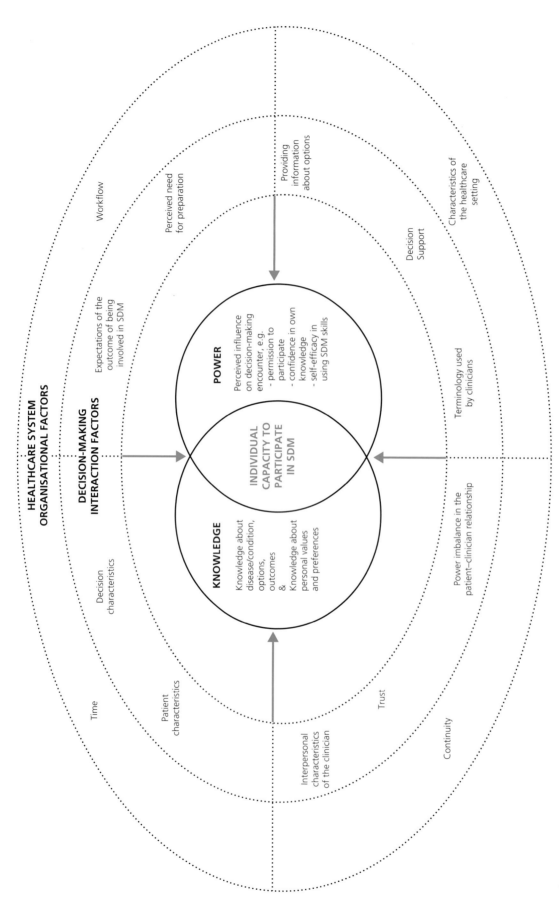

Figure 4.1 Patient-reported influences on individual capacity to participate in shared decision-making (SDM). *Source: Joseph-William et al.* (2014). Reproduced with permission of Elsevier.

HEALTHCARE SYSTEM
ORGANISATIONAL FACTORS

DECISION-MAKING
INTERACTION FACTORS

POWER

Perceived influence
on decision-making
encounter, e.g.
- permission to
participate
- confidence in own
knowledge
- self-efficacy in
using SDM skills

INDIVIDUAL
CAPACITY TO
PARTICIPATE
IN SDM

KNOWLEDGE

Knowledge about
disease/condition,
options,
outcomes
&
Knowledge about
personal values
and preferences

Workflow

Perceived need
for preparation

Providing
information
about options

Expectations of the
outcome of being
involved in SDM

Characteristics of
the healthcare
setting

Decision
Support

Decision
characteristics

Terminology used
by clinicians

Time

Patient
characteristics

Power imbalance in the
patient–clinician relationship

Interpersonal
characteristics
of the clinician

Trust

Continuity

paradigm. Barry and Edgman-Levitan (2012) express this nicely as a shift from asking, 'What is the matter?' to 'What matters to you?'

Shared decision-making has been defined as:

> An approach where clinicians and patients make decisions together using the best available evidence. Patients are encouraged to think about the available screening, treatment, or management options and the likely benefits and harms of each so that they can communicate their preferences and help select the best course of action for them. Shared decision-making respects patient autonomy and promotes patient engagement.
>
> – Elwyn *et al.* (2010)

The information exchange in shared decision-making is a natural progression and application of the definition of evidence-based medicine:

> The conscientious, explicit and judicious use of current best evidence in making decisions about the care of individual patients.
>
> – Sackett *et al.* (1996)

Shared decision-making involves placing the patient at the centre of care. It requires patients to be encouraged to express their own preferences and values, to ask questions about their care and to participate actively in the decision-making process. It requires the health professional to have the knowledge, skills and confidence to facilitate the process.

Use of shared decision-making is advocated increasingly in the use of professional guidelines. For example, in its 2014 atrial fibrillation guideline, the National Institute for Health and Care Excellence (NICE) advises discussion of the patient's preferences together with the options for anticoagulation. A series of visual decision aids, designed for patients, are provided with the guideline to facilitate discussion of risk and benefit of the various medications (see Figure 4.2).

Professional bodies increasingly provide guidance on shared decision-making. In the complex setting of end-of-life decisions the UK's General Medical Council advocates a shared model, particularly around advance care planning (see Box 4.1).

The Royal College of Surgeons of England has recently announced an educational initiative to promote shared decision-making as an attribute for its trainee surgeons. Also in the UK, the

No treatment: CHA$_2$DS$_2$-VASc score 3

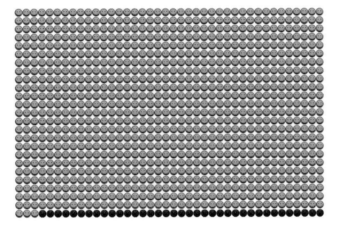

If 1000 people with AF and a CHA$_2$DS$_2$-VASc score of 3 take no anticoagulant, over 1 year on average:

- 963 people will not have an AF-related stroke (the green faces)

- 37 people will have an AF-related stroke (the red faces).

Anticoagulant: CHA$_2$DS$_2$-VASc score 3

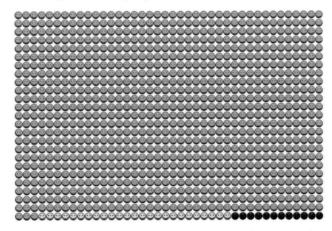

If all 1000 people take an anticoagulant, over 1 year on average:

- 963 people will not have an AF-related stroke (the green faces), but would not have done anyway

- 25 people will be saved from having an AF-related stroke (the yellow faces)

- 12 people will still have an AF-related stroke (the red faces).

Figure 4.2 Visual patient decision aid (Cates plot, www.nntonline.net) for use of an anticoagulant in the management of atrial fibrillation (AF). *Source*: Reproduced with permission of National Institute for Health and Care Excellence.

Box 4.1 **Discussion of issues in advance care planning**

- The patient's wishes, preferences or fears in relation to their future treatment and care
- The feelings, beliefs or values that may be influencing the patient's preferences and decisions
- The family members, others close to the patient or any legal proxies that the patient would like to be involved in decisions about their care
- Interventions which may be considered or undertaken in an emergency, such as cardiopulmonary resuscitation (CPR), when it may be helpful to make decisions in advance
- The patient's preferred place of care (and how this may affect the treatment options available)
- The patient's needs for religious, spiritual or other personal support

Source: Reproduced with permission of General Medical Council (2010).

Health Foundation developed and rolled out a shared decision-making programme to health professionals called MAGIC: making good decisions in collaboration (see 'Further resources').

Shared decision-making and evidence-based medicine

Evidence from research is used to determine whether an intervention, treatment or other form of management works in clinical practice. Ideally, we base decisions on synthesised high-level evidence (e.g. meta-analyses), but when not available, lower levels are used. The best possible evidence regarding the risks and benefits of a treatment are essential if shared decision-making is to produce optimal health outcomes. However use of evidence-based medicine in practice is variable, and although large population-based studies enable more rational approaches to planning and evaluation of healthcare, they can be challenging to apply to individual patients.

Although health professionals currently have more resources available to them than ever before, research suggests that only a tiny proportion of them are actually used in clinical practice. Review of medical practice in the United States suggested that care deviates from best practice about half of the time. In addition, national guidelines have high rates of non-compliance. In one study, 95% of clinicians reported awareness of lipid guidelines but followed them only 18% of the time. Similar findings have been reported in perceived and actual adherence to hypertension guidelines. Compliance with treatment is essential to improving health outcomes yet half of patients do not take their medication as directed.

The issues here are complex. If patients are to make sound decisions affecting their health they need to be presented with the available options; if the health professionals treating them are unaware of evidence, then it will be omitted from the discussion. Secondly, patients may legitimately choose not to follow best evidence due to perceived risks or harm, personal values and beliefs, or many other

individual reasons. In a particular setting, some options may not be available due to financial or other resource constraints. So, the use of evidence and shared decision-making is not straightforward. Reconciling these competing aims is assisted by considering shared decision-making as an ethical imperative, combining the four principles of autonomy, beneficence, non-maleficence and justice and thus ensuring the approach to care is centred on the patient.

Communicating information about risk

Enabling patients to make their own decisions requires health professionals to communicate information in a clear, unbiased manner. The risks and benefits of proposed treatments need to be communicated, as well as the level of uncertainty. Doing this effectively is challenging as it requires a good understanding of the situation, adequate critical appraisal skills, the ability to apply this data to the patient sitting in the consultation, and the skills to communicate in language the patient can readily understand. The health professional must recognise any bias in their own presentation of the information to the patient, which may subconsciously attempt to persuade the patient to choose a particular course of action, and account for this in the manner of the discussion with the patient. The discussion itself occurs in the context of the healthcare environment with its constraints on resources and time. In addition, the patient's understanding will be affected by personal and psychosocial perspectives resulting from prior life experience, including experiences of healthcare and the current emotions relating to the current diagnosis or stage of illness.

Strategies for encouraging shared decision-making

The responsibility for shared decision-making lies with the health professional. The patient needs to be involved from the outset of the consultation and all subsequent follow-up. The professional should know (or know how to access) the evidence base for the patient's condition or for seeking a diagnosis. The history itself should reveal the patient's perspective on their condition and particular concerns and preferences, if they are actively and deliberately sought. The professional should explain and construct a rational argument for diagnostic possibilities and actions to be taken. The reasoning process should be transparent; it should involve building rapport and maximising the quality of data gathered. These are necessary steps to enabling the patient to share decision-making. This participatory process should increase patient knowledge and autonomy, but may have an impact on consultation length and use of resources.

It is also wise to remember that shared decision-making is in the context of a complete or series of consultations. As such, the general 'atmosphere' of the consultation can facilitate or inhibit shared decision discussions. The 'four habits approach' to effective communication is a useful framework to have in mind to encourage an appropriate context, where professionals are encouraged to invest in the beginning, elicit the patient's perspective, demonstrate empathy and invest in the ending (see 'Further resources').

Combining evidence and patient preferences

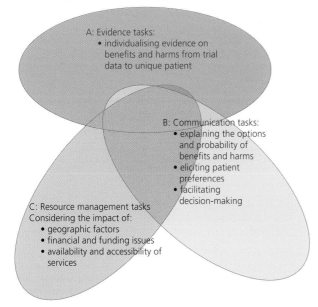

Figure 4.3 Evidence-based medicine and shared decision-making. *Source*: Barrrett (2008). Reproduced with permission of Elsevier.

Steps to shared decision-making

Shared decision-making has been described in several consultation models. Key phases may be summarised as (see also Figure 4.3):
- Listening to the patient.
- Ensuring access to good-quality evidence and information.
- Providing information tailored to the individual.
- Aiding accurate recall and understanding.
- Answering questions.
- Achieving a shared understanding.
- Ensuring patient plays an active role in the decision(s).
- Agreeing a decision (including deferral of the decision).

In their model, Elwyn *et al.* (2012) describe three types of discussion – choice, option and decision talk (see also Box 4.2):
1 Introducing *choice*.
2 Describing *options* – which may include decision support aids.
3 Helping patients make *decisions*.

Figure 4.4 illustrates the summary of the choice talk, option talk and preference talk model.

The health professional, at least in the early years of practice, or at an early stage of their own understanding of the evidence or guidelines, may rely heavily on the above models to aid the explanation. As a result of this inexperience, the discussion with the patient may not be especially individualised or contextual. Evidence may be applied in a 'heavy-handed' way to persuade patients towards a particular treatment. Guidelines are undoubtedly useful in summarising the best evidence yet they do not always take account of the patient's likely preferences – critical to the concept of shared care. Inclusion of advice for sharing decisions with patients, including the provision of decision aids, is an

increasing feature of clinical guidelines. It is clear also that a shared decision between doctor and patient, taking account of the patient's own views and interpretation of the information, will not necessarily be fully compliant with the guideline for the condition. This may be a source of concern to the practitioner, but should be viewed as both a possible and a valid consequence of a genuinely shared decision where the patient has the last say.

Presenting information to patients

In the past decade, decision aids covering a range of conditions have been developed to assist clinicians in communicating ideas of risk to patients. These aim to increase patients' understanding of the condition, the proposed treatment or treatment options and the likely benefits and risks. While the place and composition of decision aids form a growing area of research, the nonetheless certain requirements are already clear:
- Use of natural frequencies and percentages: 'If 100 patients…'.
- Use of absolute risk versus relative risk – but this is a concept that takes time to grasp.
- Framing information in a balanced manner so that risk and benefits are apparent to the patient, e.g. 'There is a risk of bleeding from your anticoagulation but we give it in order to reduce your risk of stroke'.

Box 4.2 **Summary of the choice talk, option talk and preference talk model**

Choice talk

Step back
Offer choice
Justify choice – preferences matter
Check reaction
Defer closure

Option talk

Check knowledge
List options
Describe options – explore preferences
Harms and benefits
Provide patient decision support
Summarise

Decision talk

Focus on preferences
Elicit preferences
Move to a decision
Offer review

Source: Elwyn *et al.* (2012). Reproduced with permission of Springer.

This is an open access article distributed under the terms of the Creative Commons Attribution License, which permits unrestricted use, distribution, and reproduction in any medium, provided the original work is properly cited.

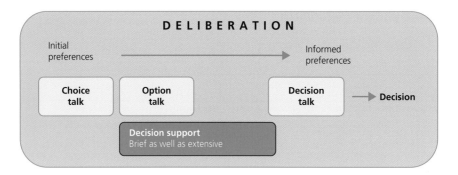

Key to the figure

Deliberation	A process where patients become aware of choice, understand their options and have the time and support to consider 'what matters most to them'; may require more than one clinical contact not necessarily face-to-face and may include the use of decision support and discussions with others.
Choice talk	Conveys awareness that a choice exists–initiated by either a patient or a clinician. This may occur before the clinical encounter.
Option talk	Patients are informed about treatment options in more detail.
Decision talk	Patients are supported to explore 'what matters most to them', having become informed.
Decision support	Decision support as designed in two formats: 1) brief enough to be used by clinician and patient together, and 2) more extensive, designed to be used by patients either before or after clinical encounters (paper, DVD, web).
Initial preferences	Awareness of options leads to the development of initial preferences, based on existing knowledge. The goal is to arrive at informed preferences.
Informed preferences	Personal preferences based on 'what matters most to patients', predicated on an understanding of the most relevant benefits and harms.

Figure 4.4 A shared decision-making model for clinical practice. *Source*: Elwyn *et al.* (2012). Reproduced with permission of Springer.

- Personalising the risk information, e.g. 'In your case, these risks don't apply, but these others do'.
- Use of graphical, pictorial or video information: these can be paper-based, online or in the form of apps.

Discussion of prognosis involves the important issue of addressing uncertainty. Patients prefer honest and accurate information and, at the same time, hope. Initiatives such as 'Wiser Choices' in the US and option grids in the UK help to convey information to patients. The Wiser Choices tools provide pictorial information combining both best evidence and patient values. So a decision aid on antidepressants combines information on 'what you need to know', weight change, sexual issues, sleep, cost, stopping and side-effects. Option grids are intended to be one-page summaries answering patients' common questions in considering treatment choices (see Figure 4.5 and Box 4.3).

The option grid can then be used to give the patient information in a structured and comprehensive manner (see Box 4.4 as an example).

Health professionals' training and development needs

Patients are increasingly likely to question the basis and evidence for their healthcare. Doctors will need to be more familiar with identifying, critiquing and using the evidence underpinning proposed treatment and management in their own speciality. They should expect patients to question the options given to them. For those patients who do not question, there is perhaps an even greater imperative to engage and inform them. There is a widening health literacy gap among some groups within our populations.

Initiatives such as the MAGIC programme in the UK encourage patients (e.g. via waiting room posters) to ask three questions during their consultation:

1 What are my options?
2 What are the benefits and harms?
3 And how likely are these?

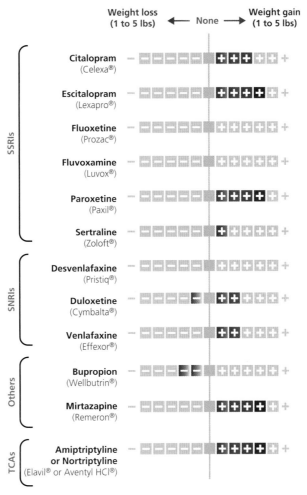

Figure 4.5 Weight changes with different antidepressants – a patient decision aid from Wiser Choices. SSRI, selective serotonin reuptake inhibitor; SNRI, serotonin–norepinephrine reuptake inhibitor; TCA, tricyclic antidepressant. *Source*: Reproduced with permission of Mayo Clinic Foundation for Research and Education.

Such initiatives may improve the quality of information sharing in the consultation (Shepherd *et al.*, 2011). They may also assist in more efficient use of time by the health professional (Montori *et al.*, 2011).

Developing the skills necessary for shared decision-making requires longitudinal training of both students and clinicians alike, not least so that students can see it role-modelled by their clinical teachers. This requires appropriate timing of the training so that students can see the skills used in a clinical context.

Training in these particular skills needs to be part of both under-graduate and postgraduate curricula. Much useful learning occurs where students actually use the skills in their own practice. Evidence-based medicine skills taught too early in the curriculum, e.g. in the preclinical years, may be lost by students by the time they reach the phase of training in which these skills may actually be useful; thus useful skills may 'atrophy' rather than develop. Similarly, actual participation in decision-making where explanation of health information and shared decision-making with patients are required and where students are able to contribute to the process, may be of greater benefit than more theoretical training at too early a stage.

Box 4.3 **Option grid for heartburn**

 U.S. English

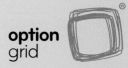

Heartburn: treatment options
Use this decision aid to help you and your healthcare professional talk about how to treat heartburn that lasts longer than 4 weeks.

Frequently Asked Questions ↓	Proton pump inhibitor medication (PPI)	Laparoscopic surgery (also known as keyhole surgery)
Why would I be offered this treatment?	If you have long-term heartburn lasting longer than 4 weeks, one possible treatment is to use medication called proton pump inhibitors (PPI)	If treatment with PPI medication is not working or giving you problems, another possible treatment is laparoscopic surgery.
What does the treatment involve?	You take one or more tablets that reduce the amount of stomach acid every day for 4 or 8 weeks, and possibly longer.	The operation makes it more difficult for acidic food to come up into the gullet (esophagus) from the stomach, and it is done under general anesthetic. It takes a week or so to recover. Medication is not usually needed after surgery.
How long will it take for the treatment to work?	Most people's symptoms improve after a few days of starting this medication.	Most people's symptoms improve soon after surgery. Swallowing might be uncomfortable for a few weeks, but this goes away.
Will my symptoms get better?	Heartburn symptoms get better in 60 to 90 in every 100 people (60–90%), but symptoms continue or come back in roughly 40 in every 100 people (40%).	Symptoms get better in 90 to 95 in every 100 people (90–95%). A small number of patients have no improvement.
What are the risks of this treatment?	Risks of serious harm are rare.	As with any surgery, there is a risk of bleeding and infection. General anesthetic can also be risky for some people. Surgery needs to be repeated in 4 to 6 in every 100 people (4–6%).
What are the side effects of this treatment?	Roughly 7 in every 100 people (7%) have side effects from the medicine. The most common mild side effects are headache, abdominal pain, nausea, diarrhea, vomiting, and increased gas.	Problems after the surgery are common, but resolve after a few days. These can include temporary difficulty in swallowing in up to 50 in every 100 people (50%), shoulder pain in roughly 60 in every 100 people (60%), and problems with belching in up to 85 in every 100 people (85%).
How long will it take me to recover from surgery?	Does not apply	Recovery takes a week or two. Most people are able to go home on the day of the operation.

Editors: Kenneth Rudd (Leaf Editor), Victoria Thomas, Mimi McCord, John de Caestecker, Marie-Anne Durand, Glyn Elwyn
Editors have declared no conflicts of interest.

Publication date: 2015-02-12 Expiry date: 2017-02-01 ISBN: 978-1-941487-03-7 License: CC BY-NC-ND 4.0 (International) This Option Grid™ decision aid does not constitute medical advice, diagnosis, or treatment. See terms of use and privacy policy at www.cptiongris.org.

Source: Reproduced with permission of the Option Grid Collaborative (http://optiongrid.org/pdf/grid/grids/56/56.en_us.1.pdf).

Box 4.4 **Shared decision-making in practice using option grids**

Case 1: A 48-year-old man with high cholesterol Concerned about a history of heart attacks in his family, a 48-year-old man asked his family doctor for a cholesterol test. It came back raised. Initially he wanted to have medication, but after reading the Option Grid with the doctor he realised that he also had to make radical changes to his lifestyle in order to reduce his risk as he was becoming aware that statins were not free of side-effects.

Case 2: A 50-year-old woman with breast cancer This patient used an Option Grid to compare mastectomy to lumpectomy (conservation surgery with radiotherapy). She noticed the difference in the local cancer recurrence rate, observing that it was double in lumpectomy. She was also alerted to the side-effects of radiotherapy, such as breast tenderness and shrinkage. These issues were important to her decision.

Case 3: A 60-year-old man with early cancer of the vocal cord Radiotherapy and surgery are both reasonable treatment options. As the patient read the Option Grid he underlined the issues for discussion. He asked about the degree and duration of hoarseness associated with radiotherapy. He emphasised that, for him, communicating with his family was of more importance than survival at any cost. The Option Grid helped to highlight his own preferences. It did so in a short time, as well as indicating the need for more detailed deliberation before making a final decision.

Source: Elwyn G *et al.* (2013). Reproduced with permission of Elsevier.

References

Barrett A. The challenge of getting both evidence and preferences into health care. Patient Educ Couns 2008; 73: 407–412.

Barry MJ, Edgman-Levitan S. Shared decision making – the pinnacle of patient-centered care. N Engl J Med 2012; 366(9): 780–781.

Elwyn G, Frosch D, Thomson R *et al*. Shared decision making: a model for clinical practice. J Gen Intern Med 2012; 27: 1361–1367.

Elwyn G, Laitner S, Coulter A *et al*. Implementing shared decision making in the NHS. Br Med J 2010; 14: 341.

Elwyn G, Lloyd A, Joseph-William N *et al*. Option Grids: shared decision making made easier. Pat Educ Couns 2013; 90: 2017–2212.

General Medical Council. Treatment and Care Towards the End of Life: Good Practice in Decision Making. UK: GMC, 2010.

Joseph-William N, Elwyn G, Edwards A. Knowledge is not power for patients: a systematic review and thematic analysis of patient-reported barriers and facilitators to shared decision making. Patient Educ Couns 2014; 94: 291–309.

Montori VM, Shah ND, Pencille LJ. Use of a decision aid to improve treatment decisions in osteoporosis: the osteoporosis choice randomized trial. Am J Med 2011; 124(6): 549–556.

Sackett DL, Rosenberg WM, Gray JA *et al*. Evidence based medicine: what it is and what it isn't? Br Med J 1996; 312: 71–72.

Shepherd HL, Barratt A, Trevena LJ *et al*. Three questions that patients can ask to improve the quality of information physicians give about treatment options: a cross-over trial. Patient Educ Couns 2011; 84(3): 379–385.

Further resources

MAGIC: shared decision making. UK: The Health Foundation. Also online: www.health.org.uk/programmes/magic-shared-decision-making. Accessed: January 2017.

Matthias MS, Salyers MP, Frankel RM. Re-thinking shared decision-making: context matters. Patient Educ Couns 2013; 91(2): 176–179.

Richard C, Lussier MT. Measuring patient participation and physician participation in exchanges on medications: dialogue ratio, preponderance of initiative, and dialogical roles. Patient Educ Couns 2007: 65; 329–341

Shay LA, Lafata JE. Where is the evidence? A systematic review of shared decision making and patient outcomes. Med Decision Making, 2015; 35(1): 114–31.

Stiggelbout AM, Van der Weigjden T, De Wit MPT *et al*. Shared decision making: really putting patients at the centre of health care. Br Med J 2012; 344: e256

CHAPTER 5

Communication in Clinical Teams

Alison Cracknell[1] and Nicola Cooper[2]

[1] Leeds Teaching Hospitals NHS Trust, Leeds, UK
[2] Derby Teaching Hospitals NHS Foundation Trust, Derby, UK

OVERVIEW

- Effective team communication reduces preventable harm.
- All members of the healthcare team should receive training in, and processes should be in place to optimise, team communication.
- Team communication in healthcare can be beset by problems, e.g. interruptions, hierarchy and a culture where people do not feel able to speak up.
- Individual training, formal handovers, safety huddles and tools like the WHO Surgical Checklist and 'time out' are ways in which team communication can be improved.
- Stating the obvious, avoiding the use of 'problematic pronouns', verbalising safety concerns and using standardised methods of communication such as SBARR are some of the ways in which individuals can communicate more effectively.

Introduction

Healthcare is increasingly complex, involving multiple clinical teams and multiple handovers of care. Healthcare teams consist of a variety of multi-professional members, with a wide range of expertise and specialist skills, and the activities of teams and their members can be widely distributed in time and location. Building effective healthcare teams can therefore be challenging and requires a continual focus and attention, not only to build, but also to maintain and enhance teamwork.

A team is not simply a group of people – it is a group of people with complimentary skills who are linked together by a common purpose in order to achieve common goals. A good team generates performance greater than the sum of its parts through synergy: team members co-ordinate their efforts and allow each member to maximise their strengths and minimise their weaknesses. Good teamwork requires that everyone communicates in a clear, effective and timely manner. Teamwork and communication in teams are among the most important skills a healthcare professional requires because it is teams, rather than individuals, who look after patients.

Effective communication is not just about providing the right information at the right time. It is also about anticipating what the risks are and the needs of others, and being mindful of the different perspectives and skills that team members bring. There is good evidence that ensuring teams communicate effectively is crucial to managing and improving patient safety, and the science of 'human factors' (see 'Further resources') emphasises team communication to enhance patient safety.

Human factors

Human factors is the science of the limitations of human performance. Increasingly, healthcare professionals are being trained in human factors and this training covers:
- the patterns and causes of error;
- the limitations of human performance;
- situation awareness and team communication.

Analysis of serious adverse events in clinical practice show that human factors, and poor team communication in particular, play a significant role when things go wrong. Contributory factors to errors in how teams function and communicate include multiple handovers, hierarchical structures and cultures that discourage challenge, and stress responses.

Situation awareness

Situation awareness involves knowing what is going on around you and being alert to potential problems. The problem is that an individual can be aware of a problem, but what is obvious to one person may not be obvious to another. A team's situation awareness can be low because no-one communicates. An example of this is shown in Box 5.1.

Team situation awareness can be compromised by:
- Poor communication
- Confusion over roles and responsibilities

ABC of Clinical Communication, First Edition. Edited by Nicola Cooper and John Frain.
© 2018 John Wiley & Sons Ltd. Published 2018 by John Wiley & Sons Ltd.

Box 5.1 **A team's situation awareness can be low because no-one communicates**

'It was obvious to everyone that things were going seriously wrong but no-one liked to mention it!'
(Quote from an air accident investigation)

'A light aircraft is heading towards an airport surrounded by mountains. The captain has inadvertently descended below the minimum safe altitude and the aircraft is on a collision course with the mountain. It is the co-pilot's first day and he can see that the aircraft is headed towards the mountain. The captain is experienced and has flown this route many times before. He is bored and preoccupied with problems at home. The co-pilot reasons that such an experienced captain surely knows what he is doing. Is there any need to say anything?'

Source: Reproduced with permission of McAllister B. Crew resource management.

Box 5.2 **Red flags**

Examples of red flags include:
- Confusion
- Conflicting or no information
- Departure from standard procedure
- Unease
- Denial or irritability
- Inaction
- Alarms
- Alarming thoughts

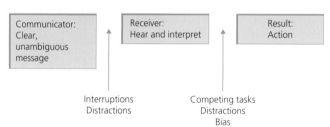

| Communicator: Clear, unambiguous message | Receiver: Hear and interpret | Result: Action |

Interruptions
Distractions

Competing tasks
Distractions
Bias

Figure 5.1 Communication has to be heard, interpreted and translated into action.

- Departure from standard procedures
- Distractions/interruptions
- Inexperience/lack of training
- Poor interpersonal skills or attitude
- Fatigue or stress.

For example, in the operating theatre there are a number of individuals all working on different aspects of patient care. They all have their own individual situation awareness.

In one imaginary scenario, a piece of tubing becomes disconnected from the ventilator. A member of theatre staff notices it, but does not think it is his place to mention it. Meanwhile, the anaesthetist notices that the patient's heart rate and blood pressure are rising. This is because the patient is receiving less anaesthetic gas; but because the anaesthetist is not aware of the disconnection, he assumes it is something else. He does not communicate his concerns to the rest of the team.

Stating what might seem obvious to you can be important. If you do not speak up, or ask for help, the team situation awareness will remain low and your own may be getting smaller and smaller as you become more stressed.

'Red flags' can be a useful means of triggering team communication. A red flag is a term we use to mean a warning. These often occur in the minutes leading up to an adverse event. Examples of red flags are shown in Box 5.2.

Look at the list in Box 5.2. Have you ever experienced a 'red flag moment'? A red flag is a cue for action. It means you have to stop to communicate with the rest of the team so that the situation can be reassessed and a decision made on how to proceed. Doing nothing is not a safe option.

Team communication

For effective communication to occur, the message needs to be clear in the first place. But often in busy healthcare environments, the message has to get through interruptions, noise and competing demands to get to the recipient. Then it has to be heard, interpreted and translated in to action (see Figure 5.1) But how do you know

that what you said will result in the intended action? The fact is that:
- What is MEANT may not be said.
- What is SAID may not be heard.
- What is HEARD may not be understood.
- What is UNDERSTOOD may not be done.

Good teams understand this is the case and take action to mitigate against it. Examples include stating the obvious (i.e. never assume that what is obvious to you is obvious to the other person); not using 'problematic pronouns' such as 'he', 'it', 'that'; and using readback – the practice of repeating back information to ensure it is correct (e.g. 'You would like me to prepare 15 – that's one five – milligrams of morphine?').

Interruptions

Team members may have different awareness of issues, and when these relate to important matters they must be verbalised and clarified, but interruptions can cause distraction and affect the flow of clinical processes as well as a person's thinking. Interruptions may contain important and essential information, e.g. an abnormal blood result that has been telephoned through, but in general interruptions should be minimised wherever possible.

Team briefings and debriefings allow time for clarifying tasks and questions and can reduce subsequent interruptions. If an interruption is necessary, if possible take the time to wait until your colleague has reached a natural break in his or her task before giving information. Likewise, if you are interrupted, acknowledge you have received the message and will deal with it next (or at an appropriate time), then finish your current task before moving on.

In clinical practice, however, emergencies always take priority over routine tasks and there will be times when you *have to* interrupt a colleague or drop everything and focus on something else instead. The ability to prioritise communication is an essential skill for any healthcare professional.

Hierarchy and culture

There is good evidence that strict hierarchies can be detrimental to patient safety, particularly if team members feel unable to speak up if they have a concern. Junior members of staff may keep quiet, assuming that experienced members of staff are fully aware of what is going on. The issue of hierarchy was clearly demonstrated in the case of Elaine Bromiley (see the case study below) – a previously healthy woman who died from hypoxic brain injury after repeated failed attempts at tracheal intubation in the anaesthetic room. Two operating theatre nurses in this case subsequently stated that they knew what needed to be done to save Elaine's life. However, they failed to assert themselves and chose indirect or passive statements, which may have been the result of the 'status asymmetry' in the room.

In some cultures, a strict hierarchy is present in healthcare organisations that is very different from what is seen, for example, in the UK. This can cause problems when people come to work in a different country, where they are expected to question when things are unclear or challenge when there are potential patient safety issues. To help people feel more comfortable in speaking out, the PACE system of raising concerns can be used, which raises concerns in a graded fashion (see Box 5.3).

Case study: Just a routine operation

Elaine Bromiley was scheduled for a routine ear, nose and throat operation. At induction of anaesthesia there were unexpected difficulties in securing her airway. In this situation the 'Can't intubate, can't ventilate' drill should have been followed. However, two

---

> Box 5.3 **PACE system of raising concerns**
>
> - Probe – ask a question, e.g. 'Do you know that…?'
> - Alert – e.g. 'I'm worried about the oxygen saturations. Can we reassess the situation for a minute?'
> - Challenge – e.g. 'Please stop what you are doing for a minute while…'
> - Emergency stop – e.g. 'STOP what you are doing!'
>
> 'PACE' teaches how to raise concerns in a graded fashion, which people feel more comfortable with. For example, one of the authors was once asked: 'Can I ask – why are you prescribing regular paracetamol for a patient who has been admitted with a paracetamol overdose?' Of course, the author had forgotten the patient with a headache had been admitted with a paracetamol overdose, and an error was averted.

---

consultant anaesthetists and an ENT surgeon struggled to secure Elaine's airway via different means for several minutes. The nurses in theatre knew what the 'Can't intubate, can't ventilate' procedure entailed and got an emergency tracheostomy kit ready and alerted the intensive care unit. However, they did not speak up. Elaine suffered hypoxic brain damage and never regained consciousness. Elaine's husband, Martin, is an airline pilot. During the course of the investigation into Elaine's death he discovered that, unlike airline staff, healthcare staff were not trained in human factors. He subsequently founded the Clinical Human Factors Group (see 'Further resources').

The official investigation into Elaine's death made the following observations:

> The management of the 'Can't intubate, can't ventilate' situation did not follow the accepted Difficult Airway Society guidelines. In particular, too much time was taken in trying to intubate the trachea rather than concentrating on ensuring adequate oxygenation by other means, such as direct access to the trachea. Whilst theatre staff ensured that all necessary equipment was available, the clinicians appeared to become oblivious to the passing of time and they lost opportunities to limit the extent of damage caused by the prolonged period of hypoxia. Given the skill mix of the clinicians, it would have been very easy to perform a surgical procedure to gain access to the trachea. Theatre staff, when interviewed, all seemed surprised that such was not performed.

The following factors critical to communication in the team were identified in the report:

- *Loss of situation awareness*. The stress of the situation meant that the consultants became highly focussed on repeated attempts to intubate the trachea. They developed 'tunnel vision' and lost track of time and the severity of the situation.
- *Teamwork*. There was no clear leader. The consultants were all helping but no one person was seen to be in charge. This led to a breakdown in the decision-making and communication between consultants.
- *Culture*. Nurses who sensed the urgency of the situation early on brought the emergency tracheostomy kit into the anaesthetic room, and alerted the intensive care unit. However, they did not raise their concerns out loud when they were not utilised. Other nurses who were aware of what was happening did not know how to broach the subject. The hierarchy of the team made assertiveness difficult despite the severity of the situation.

Optimising team communication

Team communication can be optimised by individual and team training and also having clear processes in place that facilitate good team communication. Team communication is enhanced by:

- Introducing team members
- Confirming roles and responsibilities
- Co-operating

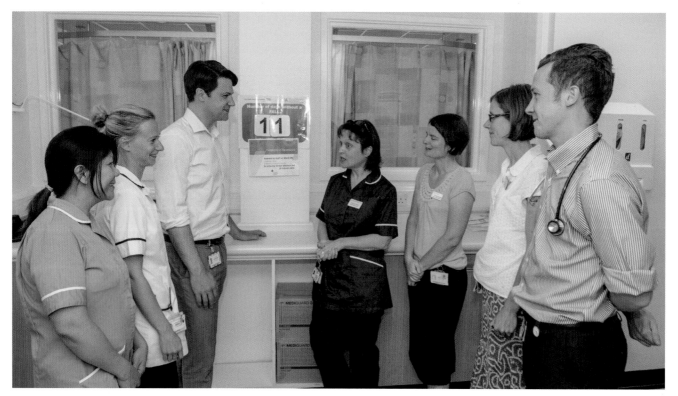

Figure 5.2 There is good evidence that team briefings and 'safety huddles' in a variety of healthcare settings can enhance teamwork and communication. Safety huddles are a recognised tool for frontline staff and caregivers.

- Reducing reliance on memory (using checklists/visual prompts)
- Listening to others
- Communicating plans clearly
- Anticipating and verbalising risks/concerns
- Asking for help if needed
- Addressing conflict.

The following are common scenarios in which team communication is often a problem, and illustrate how it can be improved.

Telephone calls

Clinicians frequently make telephone calls to other team members – to ask for advice, to refer a patient or to hand over a case. However, unstructured communication can mean that important things are missed by either party, and very often the person doing the communicating is not clear about what they want to happen next. The SBARR (situation, background, assessment, recommendation and readback) system of communicating is described in Chapter 6 and is recommended by patient safety organisations. It is particularly useful when making a phone call to a colleague when you need advice or need them to take over the care of the patient.

Handovers

Clinical handover is defined as the transfer of professional responsibility and accountability for patient care. Poor handover or failure to handover is a major cause of preventable harm. Changing work patterns and more complex care for patients mean that handover is a vital part of healthcare communication. The Royal College of Physicians of London has produced a handover toolkit with recommendations for good handovers (see Box 5.4 and Figure 5.3).

Safety huddles

There is also evidence that briefings or 'safety huddles' in a variety of healthcare settings, e.g. in-patient wards, can enhance teamwork and communication. Huddles can take many different forms. They could be part of daily briefings (e.g. before or after a ward round), part of a quality improvement intervention, or to address patient flow demands. The Institute for Healthcare Improvement has recognised huddles as a tool for frontline staff and caregivers. Figure 5.2 and Box 5.5 illustrate 'safety huddles' in action.

Emergencies

In emergencies, such as a cardiac arrest or trauma call, it is vital that there is a team leader and everyone knows who that is. This ensures clarity of communication during what can be a stressful period for members of the team. Ideally, each team member has an allocated role in advance. For example, modern trauma team members wear tabards that clearly identify their role ('team leader', 'anaesthetist' or 'runner') but if not, the team leader should delegate roles clearly. It is important to verbalise your actions during an emergency so that everyone else knows what you are doing. This avoids accidental duplication or misunderstanding. (e.g. '1 mg adrenaline being administered now'). If you are called to an emergency, first clarify

Out of hour handover (please complete in block capitals)

Handover details

Handed over by _____   Handed over to _____

Day(s) covered by this handover (please circle)   Mon   Tue   Weds   Thu   Fri   Sat   Sun

Patient surname, forename date of birth, NHS hospital no	Responsible consultant, patient current location	Diagnosis/problem list/ differential diagnosis (include any risks or warnings)	Reason for handover	Outstanding issues (tasks to be done)	Aims and limitations of treatment (e.g. resus/ITU/ventilation/inotropes/active/ palliative/surgery–yes/no)
					Weekend discharge yes/no
					Weekend discharge yes/no
					Weekend discharge yes/no
					Weekend discharge yes/no
					Weekend discharge yes/no

Figure 5.3 Example handover sheet.

Box 5.4 **Royal College of Physicians recommendations for handover (see 'Further resources')**

Effective handovers should:
- Be tailored to the local unit/department
- Define who must be present
- Occur at a designated time and place
- Standardise an order of proceedings
- Use a standard system for communicating
- Determine clear arrangements for the ongoing care of patients
- Determine the immediacy of review and by whom
- Be documented.

There should also be training in team communication and handover at the start of a new post (induction).

Box 5.5 **Safety huddles in action**

Safety huddles on wards at the Leeds Teaching Hospitals NHS Trust consist of a daily patient safety meeting about one or more agreed patient harms (which the team have decided to focus on) such as falls, pressure ulcers and avoidable deterioration. The safety huddle is a short meeting (5–10 minutes) that takes place daily at an agreed time and location on the ward and involves all members of the healthcare team, including non-clinical staff (e.g. housekeepers and ward clerks).

The meeting follows some general principles: staff review how many days it is since the last fall, cardiac arrest (or other agreed harm), and look at who may be at risk of the harm today and what actions need to be implemented by the team to reduce that risk. The meetings are non-hierarchical and everyone is encouraged to raise any concerns or make suggestions. When a harm or incident has occurred since the last huddle, the whole team debriefs, learns what the contributory factors were, and the learning is communicated to the wider team.

These huddles have been associated with reductions in harm, including falls, pressure ulcers, medication delays and overall improvements in the ward safety culture.

Wards choose for themselves exactly how they want to introduce safety huddles and which harm(s) they want to focus on. Posters that record the days since the last harm event and improvement run charts are displayed and used in the huddle. Certificates are also provided for wards that achieve significant milestones in days since the last harm event.

---

who is in charge. Ideally, this person should not perform any other role apart from directing the team, listening to their concerns, and co-ordinating the patient's care.

WHO surgical checklist

The World Health Organization Safe Surgery checklist and 'time out' is an example of how simple solutions can optimise team communication, minimise hierarchy and reduce error (Figure 5.4).

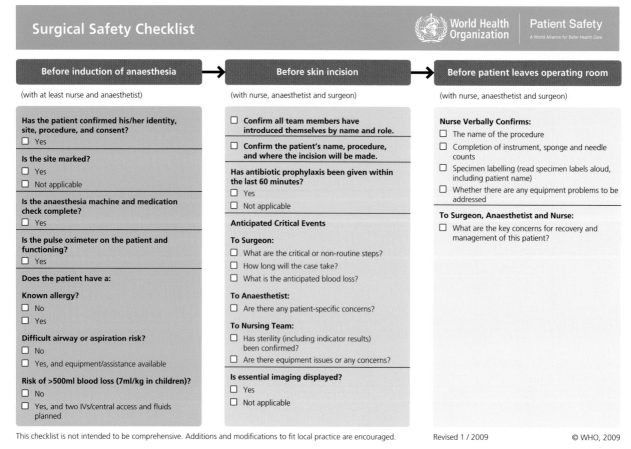

Figure 5.4 WHO Surgical Safety Checklist. *Source:* Reproduced with permission of World Health Organization (2008).

All team members must introduce themselves, confirm roles, confirm essential patient and procedure details, as well as plan and anticipate critical events during a team briefing prior to the start of the operating list. The use of the WHO Surgery Checklist during the operating list (including a 'time out' before each case in which every team member has to agree the patient's identity and the procedure to be performed) reduced mortality and surgical complications by more than one-third across eight pilot hospitals. The rate of major in-patient complications dropped from 11% to 7%, and the in-patient death rate following major surgery fell from 1.5% to 0.8% (see 'Further resources').

Conclusions

Effective communication and optimal teamwork reduce preventable harm. All members of the healthcare team should receive training in team communication, and systems should be in place to optimise this (e.g. handovers, safety huddles, 'time outs' in theatre). Team members should confirm their roles and responsibilities, anticipate, co-operate, verbalise concerns, listen to others, give clear instructions and ask for help. Ideally, teams that work together should also train together.

References

McAllister B. Crew Resource Management. Awareness, Cockpit Efficiency and Safety. Shrewsbury, UK: Airlife Publishing, 1997.

World Health Organization. WHO Surgical Safety Checklist and Implementation Manual, 2008. Online: http://www.who.int/patientsafety/safesurgery/ss_checklist/en/ (open access): Accessed: May 2017.

Further resources

Clinical Human Factors Group: www.chfg.org. Accessed: October 2016. You can see a video that reconstructs the Elaine Bromiley case at https://youtu.be/JzlvgtPIof4 and the anonymised incident investigation report is freely available on the Internet with the family's permission.

Cooper N. Human factors. In: Cooper N, Frain J (eds). ABC of Clinical Reasoning. Oxford: Wiley, 2016.

Gordon S, Mendenhall P, O'Connor BB. Beyond the Checklist: What Else Healthcare Can Learn from Aviation Teamwork and Safety. ILR Press, 2012.

Haynes AB, Weiser TG, Berry WR *et al.* A surgical safety checklist to reduce morbidity and mortality in a global population. N Engl J Med 2009; 360: 491–499.

Royal College of Physicians. Acute Care Toolkit 1: Handover. London, UK: RCP, 2015. https://www.rcplondon.ac.uk/guidelines-policy/acute-care-toolkit-1-handover. Accessed: May 2017.

Vincent C. Patient Safety, 2nd edn. Oxford, UK: Wiley-Blackwell, 2010.

CHAPTER 6

Communication in Medical Records

Nigel D.C. Sturrock

Derby Teaching Hospitals NHS Foundation Trust, Derby, UK

> **OVERVIEW**
>
> - The entries you make in medical records should be accurate, concise, legible, ideally written contemporaneously, signed, dated and timed.
> - As well as contributing to case management, the medical records can be used to determine mortality statistics, contribute to audit, influence payment and be referred to in legal and inquest cases.
> - Medical records are confidential and must be kept secure, accessed only by clinicians involved in the case, and if used for broader purposes they should be anonymised with only the minimum data required divulged.
> - It is the duty of the responsible clinician to ensure that there is a satisfactory handover of relevant clinical information to the next team; this also includes during transfer of care to another provider.
> - Electronic patient records (EPRs) provide advantages to paper records given the opportunities to improve accuracy and ensure no omissions, offering wider accessibility to enhance shared decision-making; but EPRs are not without issues, such as the need to maintain security and confidentiality.

It is said that, 'If it isn't written in the notes, it did not happen.' While this is obviously incorrect, what this statement highlights is that if something is documented in the medical records it is taken as proof that it did happen. Accurate medical notes are therefore not only an important means to managing a patient's case, acting as a record of the diagnoses and action plans from the history, physical examination and investigation results, but they are also an effective means of communication between healthcare professionals involved in the case, and, in addition, provide a log of what was done and why. This chapter will consider the many facets of medical note-keeping as well as providing some simple tips on good communication in medical records.

General Medical Council perspective

In the UK, the General Medical Council's document *Good Medical Practice* (see Figure 6.1) describes that clinical records must be clear, accurate and legible, and ideally completed contemporaneously. The record should contain the relevant clinical findings, management plans and actions, and should identify which clinicians are involved in the case and what information was given to patients.

The GMC expects that every doctor registered with them and holding a licence to practice should have an annual appraisal of their practice, and on a 5-yearly basis submit evidence of good medical practice to support their revalidation. The appraisal process may include aspects of medical note-keeping. An audit tool on clinical standards for medical record-keeping has been produced by the Royal College of Physicians of London (see 'Further resources').

The National Health Service code of practice

Medical records are confidential and must be stored securely and meet local information governance policies. Clinicians are expected to maintain the confidentiality of medical records of their patients, but at the same time to share relevant information with other clinicians involved in the patient's care.

Dame Fiona Caldicott developed principles in relation to the sharing of personally identifiable information in 1997 (known as the 'Caldicott principles'). These were revised in 2013 and consist of the following principles that cover many fields of practice in healthcare, including carrying out audits or research studies or simply being asked to provide information about a patient to the Police. You must:
- Be aware of your responsibilities.
- Justify the purpose for sharing.

ABC of Clinical Communication, First Edition. Edited by Nicola Cooper and John Frain.
© 2018 John Wiley & Sons Ltd. Published 2018 by John Wiley & Sons Ltd.

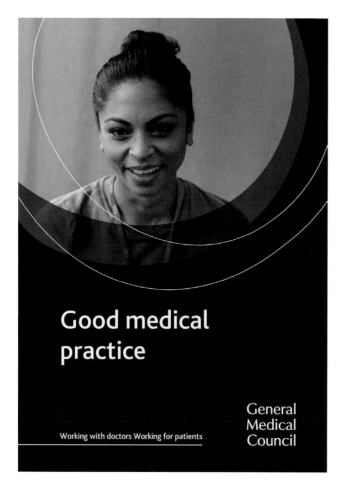

Figure 6.1 The UK General Medical Council's *Good Medical Practice* (2013) outlines four domains of practice: knowledge, skills and performance; safety and quality; communication, partnership and teamwork; and maintaining trust. The domain of communication, partnership and teamwork is assessed on a regular basis for all doctors with a licence to practice in the UK through various means, e.g. work-based assessments (for doctors in training), 360° colleague feedback, patient satisfaction surveys and compliments/complaints received. *Source*: General Medical Council UK (open access).

- Not use personally identifiable information unless it is absolutely necessary.
- Use the minimum personally identifiable information.
- Access personally identifiable information on a strict need-to-know basis.
- Understand and comply with the law, e.g. the UK's Data Protection Act.
- Understand that the duty to share information can be as important as the duty to protect patient confidentiality.

If you are ever in doubt, you should inform your local 'Caldicott Guardian' about the issue and seek their advice on what information you can share (see Box 6.1).

The UK's Health and Social Care Information Centre (now called 'NHS Digital') produced guidance in 2013: a guide to confidentiality in health and social care (see 'Further resources') It outlined five 'rules' to advise clinicians:

1 Information about service users or patients should be treated confidentially and respectfully.

Box 6.1 **Caldicott Guardians**

A 40-year-old commercial airline pilot was admitted to the general hospital following an episode of transient loss of consciousness that sounded like syncope. He stated it was because he had been particularly tired following a period of stress at home and did not think it would be a problem in the future. He did not want to inform his employer about it.

He had no past medical history, and his physical examination, blood tests and 12-lead electrocardiogram were all normal.

The doctors were unsure as to whether they could disclose this information against his will to his employers, and sought the advice of their local Caldicott Guardian.

A Caldicott Guardian is a senior person, for example a medical director, who is responsible for protecting the confidentiality of patient and service-user information and at the same time enabling lawful and appropriate information-sharing. Health and social care organisations that access patient records in the UK are required to have a Caldicott Guardian.

---

2 Members of a care team should share confidential information when it is needed for the safe and effective care of an individual.
3 Information that is shared for the benefit of the community should be anonymised.
4 An individual's right to object to the sharing of confidential information about them should be respected.
5 Organisations should put policies, procedures and systems in place to ensure the confidentiality rules are followed.

As a result, healthcare organisations require all their staff to undergo information governance training and this is usually updated on an annual basis. The training covers all aspects of information governance and your role and responsibilities in relation to medical records and personal information (see Figure 6.2 and Box 6.2).

Medical note-keeping and mortality data

Within the UK's National Health Service, mortality statistics are seen as an important albeit blunt measure of one aspect of quality of care. Increasingly, across surgical and medical specialities, an individual clinician's mortality data are being published for patients to access. Mortality statistics are constructed using the observed versus the expected death rate. Data that impact on the calculation of the expected death rate relate to the complexity of a patient's condition and the number of other contributory medical conditions. A number of co-morbidities derived from the *International Classification of Diseases* (ICD) codes are considered particularly relevant, and are given a weighting score, based on the adjusted risk of death and resource use, which when summed together give the Charlson Co-morbidity Index for a patient and the episode of care (see Box 6.3).

It is therefore in the interests of the clinician, as an individual as well as for the organisation they work for, that all co-morbidities are accurately recorded in the medical notes, so that the correct Charlson Co-morbidity Index is calculated and the correct expected mortality rate derived.

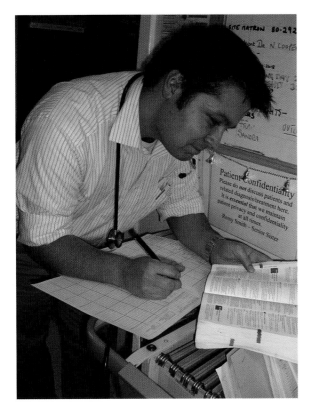

Figure 6.2 Take care when talking in public places.

Box 6.2 **Information governance training**

Information governance training usually uses scenarios to help people learn about how to look after and keep information confidential. Typical scenarios might include the following:
- Use of unencrypted memory sticks to store identifiable patient data
- A patient requesting to see their hospital notes
- Two doctors talking loudly about a case in the canteen
- Taking hospital notes home to finish an audit
- Giving a colleague your IT password
- Being asked about a person's diagnosis by a police officer
- Looking up the results of a celebrity who has been admitted to your hospital.

Box 6.3 **The Charlson Co-morbidity Index**

The Charlson Co-morbidity Index predicts 1-year mortality for a patient with a range of co-morbid conditions (a total of 22 conditions). Each condition is assigned a score of 1, 2, 3 or 6 depending on the risk of dying associated with each one. The total score is used to predict mortality. Many variations of this score have also been produced.

Score	Comorbid condition
1 each	Myocardial infarction (history, not ECG changes alone)
	Congestive cardiac failure
	Peripheral vascular disease (including aortic aneurysm)
	Dementia
	Cerebrovascular disease (TIA or stroke with no/minimal residual signs)
	Chronic lung disease
	Connective tissue disease
	Peptic ulcer disease
	Mild liver disease (without portal hypertension)
	Diabetes without end-organ damage (excluding diet-controlled alone)
2 each	Hemiplegia
	Moderate or severe kidney disease
	Diabetes with end-organ damage
	Tumour without metastasis (excluding if at least 5 years since diagnosis)
	Leukaemia (acute or chronic)
	Lymphoma
3	Moderate or severe liver disease
6 each	Metastatic solid tumour
	AIDS (not just HIV-positive)

In the original study the 1-year mortality rates for the different scores were:
- Zero: 12%
- 1–2: 26%
- 3–4: 52%
- ≥5: 85%

Source: Charlson *et al.* (1987). Reproduced with permission of Elsevier.

Medical note-keeping and payment

In the same way that the complexity of a patient's medical condition impacts on the expected mortality rate, so the complexity of a patient's condition and the types of procedures performed on them influence the payment that is given to the hospital in many countries' healthcare systems. The medical records are used as the basis to code the complexity of the case as well as all the procedures that were carried out during the episode of care. Medical diagnoses derive from ICD codes. If there are any omissions in the notes, or if medical conditions are not clearly documented and/or code-able (e.g. writing 'acute confusion', which is not a medical diagnosis

instead of 'delirium', which is) then whether it be a clinical condition or a procedure, it cannot be coded and therefore paid for, even if it existed or happened. Thus, how clearly clinicians document medical diagnoses and existing co-morbidities in the notes has a direct effect on their organisation's financial well-being.

In the UK, a hospital's coding department codes medical diagnoses from the notes to process episodes of care for payment. Coders can code an entry in the notes that begins with 'diagnosis', 'treat as', 'probably', 'presumed', as well as from symptoms where no definite diagnosis is made. However, they cannot code anything that starts with 'query' or '?', 'differential diagnosis', 'possible', 'likely' or 'suspected'. If, on discharge, histology is awaited for a definitive diagnosis then this should be noted.

It is also important to avoid the use of ambiguous abbreviations. For example, 'M.S.' could mean multiple sclerosis or mitral stenosis; 'P.I.D' could mean prolapsed intervertebral disc or pelvic inflammatory disease. If a clear diagnosis has not been reached, make sure you detail the main symptoms in the notes or discharge summary instead.

Simple tips for good medical note-keeping

Although this section describes advice when writing in paper notes, many of the principles are applicable to electronic medical records as well. It is important to do the following:

- Write clearly and legibly in the notes and on discharge documentation, using black ink only (other colours do not photocopy well, which can be important later in legal case/inquests).
- Make sure the patient is identified on every sheet of paper used in the notes.
- Sign, date and time every entry in the notes. Print your name and position at the end of every entry.
- Write in the notes contemporaneously or as soon as possible after patient contact.
- If you need to add something to a medical record or make a correction, make sure you enter the date of the amendment and include your name. You must draw a single line through the part that you wish to correct and must *never* remove pages or obliterate a previous entry so it can no longer be read.
- Clearly record details of all the diagnoses (including co-morbidities) and procedures in the notes.
- For injuries, note the cause; for overdoses, note the drug; and for infections, note the organism.
- If you are a trainee, ask a senior member of the medical staff to confirm or validate diagnoses and procedures.
- Include the details of all diagnoses and procedures on discharge summaries.
- Never use pejorative terms.
- Never remove medical notes from your place of work.

Letters and discharge summaries

There is an art to writing a well-constructed referral or clinic letter or discharge summary. Mandated fields on electronic templates are aimed at ensuring that critical information is not inadvertently missed out. How those fields are filled out, however, is important. Avoid long rambling narratives – clinicians are working under pressure and need to read correspondence quickly; critical information may be buried and go unnoticed. Think in advance about the important information you wish to convey and then write it in a concise matter. This will result in a letter that is appreciated by the recipient (see Box 6.4).

The UK's General Medical Council states that the clinician ordering a test is responsible for checking its result and acting on it once available. It is not appropriate to request outpatient investigations and then expect someone else (e.g. the general practitioner) to chase the results and act on them. It is, however, acceptable to give advice on further management that might include suggestions to check a blood test or increase the dose of a new medication later.

Box 6.4 Template for concise discharge summaries and clinic letters

Discharge letter	Clinic letters
Name and hospital number	Clinic date
	Name and hospital number
Date of admission	Diagnosis list
Date of discharge	4. a
Diagnosis list	5. b
1. a	6. c etc
2. b	Any action for GP (including medication changes)
3. c etc	Follow-up
Medications (and changes)	Dear Doctor, (Include what you think about the possible diagnosis and where you are heading in terms of management – this makes it easier for colleagues who see the patient after you)
Allergies	
Follow-up	
Any action for GP	
Dear Doctor,	
(Brief summary)	

Help the secretary and the reader by being concise. This is no need to dictate 'this 70-year-old man was admitted with a cough, breathlessness and fever and his test results showed raised white cells and right lower zone consolidation on the chest x-ray....' when you can say 'Mr X was admitted with pneumonia'.

Source: Courtesy of Cooper *et al.* (2006). Reproduced with permission of BMJ-Blackwell.

It is also standard practice to give patients a copy of their clinical letter or discharge summary; therefore consider whether the text is understandable for laypeople and whether the patient and/or their relatives are aware of any sensitive information that may be included.

Legal aspects of medical note-keeping

No matter how good a clinician you are and how diligent you may be, inevitably in clinical practice things can go wrong. Whether it is a complaint from a patient, a negligence claim or a Coroner's Inquest (Procurator Fiscal in Scotland), the contemporaneous notes provide a critical source of information to defend your actions. Given that patients, family members and lawyers can all legitimately request access to the full set of medical records pertaining to the issue of concern, as a clinician the standard of your medical note-keeping and your professionalism will be under scrutiny.

Multidisciplinary records

Increasingly, medical, nursing and other professionals use the same healthcare record, and there is a growing recognition that for many patients, a multidisciplinary team is required to manage their condition. As such, sharing of and access to important clinical information

Use the SBARR system of communicating!

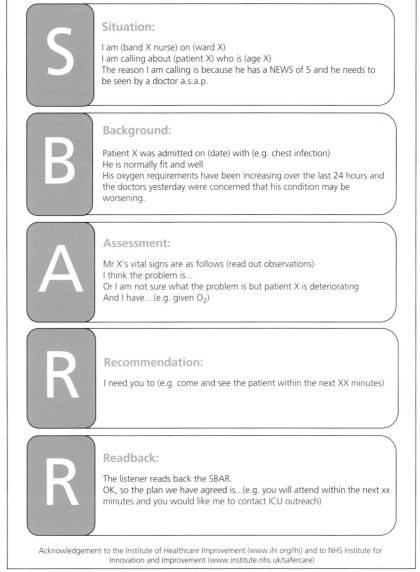

Situation:

I am (band X nurse) on (ward X)
I am calling about (patient X) who is (age X)
The reason I am calling is because he has a NEWS of 5 and he needs to be seen by a doctor a.s.a.p.

Background:

Patient X was admitted on (date) with (e.g. chest infection)
He is normally fit and well
His oxygen requirements have been increasing over the last 24 hours and the doctors yesterday were concerned that his condition may be worsening.

Assessment:

Mr X's vital signs are as follows (read out observations)
I think the problem is...
Or I am not sure what the problem is but patient X is deteriorating
And I have...(e.g. given O_2)

Recommendation:

I need you to (e.g. come and see the patient within the next XX minutes)

Readback:

The listener reads back the SBAR.
OK, so the plan we have agreed is...(e.g. you will attend within the next xx minutes and you would like me to contact ICU outreach)

Acknowledgement to the Institute of Healthcare Improvement (www.ihi.org/ihi) and to NHS Institute for Innovation and Improvement (www.institute.nhs.uk/safercare)

SBARR has been shown to improve the effectiveness of communication and takes less time.

Figure 6.3 The SBARR communication tool.

is an important aspect of clinical governance, and one enabler of this is a single clinical record that all multidisciplinary team members contribute to contemporaneously. This minimises duplication, improves accuracy and clarity by maintaining focus on relevant clinical details, and can support effective sharing of information.

Medical notes as a handover tool

Handover of care from one clinical team to another is an everyday occurrence, but if not done properly it can be a major contributory factor to error and patient harm. The UK's Academy of Medical Royal Colleges has produced guidance on the content of handover sheets (see 'Further resources').

Acronyms have also been devised to prompt clinicians with a checklist of the elements of effective verbal communication at

> **Box 6.5 SHOP – a template for team handover**
>
> - Sick – which patients are most ill
> - Home – which patients are ready for discharge
> - Others – a round-up of the rest of the patients
> - Plan – how the work should be divided/prioritised

handover. These can be incorporated in to handover sheets. SBARR is a commonly used one (see Figure 6.3) and SBARR handover sheets can be found in many hospitals; SHOP is another (see Box 6.5). Remember that handover sheets contain patient identifiable data and must be kept confidential at all times.

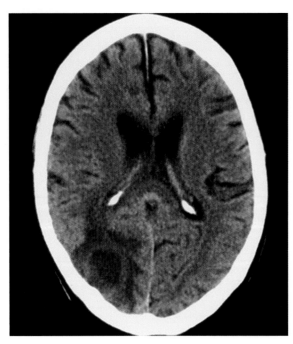

Figure 6.4 Picture archiving communication systems (PACS) are also medical records – do not leave screens open for unauthorised people to view.

Electronic patient records

In its broadest sense, electronic patient records include results servers and things like the Picture Archiving Communication System (PACS), used by many hospitals to store and view radiological investigations (see Figure 6.4). There are a number of other software systems that healthcare organisations use for electronic patient/health records. One example of this is the summary care record (SCR). This record consists of information about a patient's current medications and allergies. Data-sharing agreements between organisations allow clinical teams, often in emergency departments or assessment units, to access the SCR, ensuring that medication errors are minimised.

Inevitably there are downsides to such systems. They must be encrypted, and only appropriate users involved in the care of a patient should be able to access what might be highly sensitive information. One issue is that once users have access to a system, they can look at any record on the system. It is therefore critical that they are made fully aware of their obligations not to misuse the system via appropriate training on all aspects of information governance.

Personal held records

Well-informed patients are often best placed to manage their own health. As such, having access to their own information in understandable terminology, with an interpretation of what the diagnoses and results mean is important. This can be particularly pertinent for patients with long-term conditions or cancer, as well as during pregnancy. The personal held record (PHR) has still not been widely applied across the National Health Service but systems are available in digital format with access through online portals, allowing patients to access their own medical records, add to them, organise them and integrate them with records held by a variety of healthcare providers. There needs to be a cultural and behavioural shift for the PHR to become widely used, as well as a need to fully inform patients of the benefits and risks of the PHR as well as training on how to access and use it to its maximum potential.

Conclusions

It is incumbent on all clinicians to ensure that the entries in medical records clearly identify the author, have a time/date stamp on each entry, reflect objectively the findings, contribute constructively to the management of the case, and are kept confidential and secure.

References

Charlson ME, Pompei P, Ales KL, MacKenzie CR. A new method of classifying prognostic comorbidity in longitudinal studies: development and validation. J Chron Dis 1987; 40: 373–383.

Cooper N, Forrest K, Cramp P, eds. Essential Guide to Generic Skills. Oxford, UK: BMJ-Blackwell, 2006.

General Medical Council. Good Medical Practice. London, UK: GMC, 2013.

Further resources

Academy of Medical Royal Colleges. A Clinician's Guide to Record Standards. Parts 1 and 2. London, UK: AoMRC, 2008.

BMA Junior Doctors' Committee. Safe Handover: Safe Patients. Guidance on Clinical Handover for Clinicians and Managers. London, UK: BMA, 2004.

Department of Health. Information: To share or not to share? The information governance review. London, UK: DoH, 2013 (also known as the 'Caldicott review'). Online: https://www.gov.uk/government/publications/the-information-governance-review. Accessed: May 2017.

Health and Social Care Information Centre. A Guide to Confidentiality In Health And Social Care. London, UK: HSCIC, 2013.

Royal College of Physicians of London. Generic Medical Record Keeping Standards. London, UK: RCP, 2009. Online: https://www.rcplondon.ac.uk/projects/outputs/generic-medical-record-keeping-standards. Accessed: May 2017.

CHAPTER 7

Advanced Communication for Specific Situations

Nivedita Aswani, Vanessa Cox and Julia Surridge

Derbyshire Children's Hospital, Derby, UK

OVERVIEW

- The typical doctor–patient consultation can be challenging at times for a variety of reasons – for example, the patient could be a child or young person, they may be angry, have a chronic illness, or there may be safeguarding issues that should be explored.

- Some useful frameworks and techniques are outlined in this chapter to deal with such situations, e.g. the 'HEADSSS assessment' for young people or motivational interviewing for patients with chronic illnesses.

- Difficult consultations will not always proceed according to the doctor's agenda, and flexibility in communication style and techniques is required.

- It is useful to reflect on the learning from difficult conversations in order to build skills and confidence in such situations.

Paediatric consultations

Children and young people are almost always seen accompanied by a parent or carer during a medical consultation. Three common exceptions to this include:

- A medical interview where there are safeguarding concerns and the young person is of an age to speak independently and able to make disclosures.
- A young person with a chronic illness in the transition process to adult care.
- A teenager with risk-taking behaviour who has presented unaccompanied, or was brought in by school or friends to the emergency department.

Aside from such situations, the paediatric interview is usually a 'triadic consultation' between health professional, young person and at least one parent or carer. This poses unique challenges. Families vary in their views regarding the extent to which the encounter should be child-centred, and therefore the doctor needs to actively support the young person's involvement to avoid an exclusive doctor–adult dyad. Involving both patient and carer to their mutual satisfaction is a difficult skill to accomplish.

Consider the four main parts of a consultation:

- Introductions
- Information-gathering
- Treatment-planning
- Discussion.

Children are often only involved in the initial social introductions to put them at ease and gain their trust. During information-gathering, although carers are more likely to have accurate details of birth, developmental and past medical history, and while their concerns, observations and theories are valid, always make an effort to allow children to describe symptoms in their own language and to tell you how they are affected by them through open questioning. Exploring their theories on aetiology can be enlightening and reveal worries that their carers may be unaware of. Talking to them directly may encourage a disclosure of important information which may not otherwise come to light. Children also need to be given the opportunity to take part in decision-making around treatment. Expression of their views and seeking their consent should take place wherever possible, taking into account their level of understanding and competence. A scenario to illustrate this is seen in Figure 7.1.

Difficult behaviours: the angry or violent patient

Consider the case history in Box 7.1. This is a common scenario in which a clinician's professional opinion is either at odds with the family/patient's beliefs (e.g. that they don't believe in giving their child medicine) or at odds with their opinion (e.g. that they need a prescription to make it better). It is important to explore anger – in this scenario, you have been given an insight into why this mother is so angry. This is explored more in a further triadic conversation model in Figure 7.2.

The following is a useful way to proceed:

- Listen to the mother and make sure that your body language is non-threatening. Breaking eye contact intermittently is useful, focusing on the child and smiling at her.

ABC of Clinical Communication, First Edition. Edited by Nicola Cooper and John Frain.
© 2018 John Wiley & Sons Ltd. Published 2018 by John Wiley & Sons Ltd.

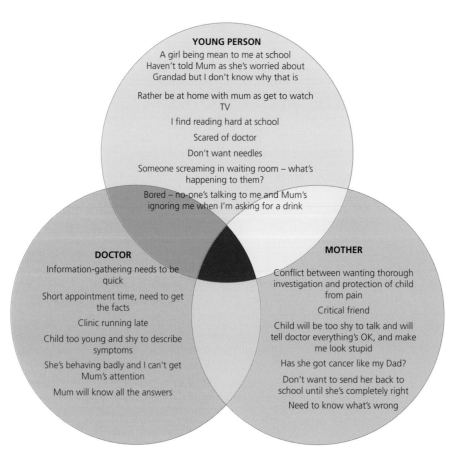

Figure 7.1 The triadic consultation. A 9-year-old girl is referred by her general practitioner for recurrent bouts of abdominal pain, causing poor school attendance. The girl's mother suffers from chronic back pain with limited mobility, and her paternal grandfather has just been diagnosed with pancreatic cancer. What is going on in everyone's mind? Unless the doctor is skilled and vigilant in involving both parties, their agendas and information may remain hidden, and leave one or more parties dissatisfied.

Box 7.1 **Case history: difficult behaviours**

A mother and grandmother attended the general practice surgery with a 2½-year-old child who had been hot, miserable and had ulcers in her mouth. The ulcers appeared 5 days ago and since then the child has worsened, and was now not eating or drinking well.

On examination, the child was not clinically dehydrated, had a low-grade fever of 37.8°C and had multiple ulcers throughout her mouth consistent with herpes gingivostomatitis. There were no other examination features of concern. However, during the physical examination the mother's body language became increasingly hostile.

The doctor asked questions to confirm that appropriate and regular pain relief had been given. The mother questioned whether she was being accused of neglecting her daughter by not given her pain medicine. The grandmother stated it was 'impossible' as the child just spat it out. The mother became increasingly angry, stating she had not slept and was in a lot of pain herself due to her own medical problems. 'Doctors always blame things on viruses when they don't know what the problem is and can't do anything,' she said.

How should you proceed, and at what point in the discussion should you explain that there is no specific treatment for this condition?

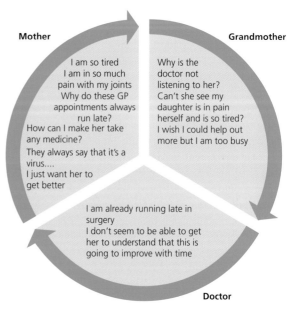

Figure 7.2 Angry family consultation: triadic conversation.

- Acknowledge the mother's concerns and show empathy – e.g. frustration at not being able to give medication, tiredness, how unpleasant it is to see your child in pain.
- Ask an open question such as, 'You seem very angry – why is that?' This should allow the mother to explain what has happened and gives you an 'in' to the conversation. Be prepared for angry responses, but remember it is the mother who is angry, not you.
- Acknowledge the limitations of medicine on occasions. This is an opportunity to explain the pathophysiology of the condition, e.g. ulcers can progress for up to a week but then the pain significantly improves.
- Acknowledge her attempts at giving medication appropriately and offer advice on how to do it. Consider adding something such as an anaesthetic mouth spray to assist with giving oral medication.
- Emphasise how common this condition is, and that it is very rare to require hospitalisation, continuing to emphasise that the girl is not dehydrated because the family have clearly been doing all the right things.
- Summarise your findings and reasons for the diagnosis that you have made. Summarise the treatment points and emphasise again the important or regular analgesia.
- Allow time for questions.

Language barriers

When there are language barriers, efforts must be made to provide face-to-face interpreters from a reputable agency, speaking the appropriate language and dialect of the patient. This is another form of triadic communication; however, in this instance, it is difficult to verify the exact information that is being transferred, and steps should be taken to make sure you have faith in the dialogue being translated accurately (see Box 7.2).

If you can, avoid using the following in lieu of an interpreter:
- Family members or friends
- Telephone language services
- Children under 18 years of age
- Untrained volunteers
- Other patients or visitors
- Internet translation sites.

Be aware of the fact that if you are breaking bad news, an interpreter may try to ease the distress of the patient by withholding upsetting information. It may be the case that the interpreter lives in the same close-knit ethnic community, so the patient may be reluctant to disclose sensitive information. If you have any concerns about the integrity or skills of a professional interpreter, contact their agency and do not use them again.

An inability to speak English will also mean that the patient is unlikely to be able to read written communication from the hospital, so take the opportunity to use the interpreter to ensure the patient is aware of the next appointment date and time. Check the patient's address and contact details and the best methods for communicating future appointments and care plans. Explore any other reasons why the person may find it difficult to access health care.

> **Box 7.2 Tips for communicating effectively using interpreters**
>
> - Introduce yourself to the interpreter.
> - Give clear instructions to the interpreter about translating your dialogue directly *without* their own interpretation.
> - Give clear expectations to the interpreter about respecting patient confidentiality and check that the patient is aware that sensitive issues may need to be discussed.
> - Be vigilant to clues about quality of interpretation (e.g. shortening of a long dialogue from the doctor into a brief sentence to the patient, and vice versa). However, some words or concepts do not have a direct literal translation into every other language, and this may take longer than your original speech.
> - Verify the passage of information by questioning the interpreter directly.
> - Speak and give eye contact to the patient, not the interpreter.
> - Speak slowly rather than loudly.
> - Avoid confusing the need for interpretation with poor cognition; however, at the same time, effective interpretation does not necessarily imply understanding and this must be verified.
> - Speak at a slow pace and break down dialogue into small segments with sufficient pauses to ensure the interpreter can translate everything you say.
> - Insist that everything you, and the patient says, is translated.
> - Allow the patient adequate time to ask their own questions.
> - Ask the patient to repeat back important information and encourage the interpreter to alert you if they do not feel the patient understands.

Exploring safeguarding concerns

Safeguarding relates to the promotion of welfare of children and adults in order to protect them from harm. Safeguarding is everyone's responsibility, and any professional who has a concern about an individual's welfare should make a referral to the appropriate agency, or at the very least discuss it with their immediate line manager. Relevant organisations (e.g. health and social care, schools and the police) and clinicians must collaborate effectively, and it is therefore vital that every individual working with children and families or vulnerable adults is aware of their own role and that of other professionals in terms of safeguarding. Figure 7.3 outlines some of the common categories of abuse that require safeguarding actions.

Several principles apply to safeguarding:
- It is mandatory for clinicians working in the UK to undertake the appropriate level of safeguarding training
- Think of safeguarding issues, or non-accidental injury, as a differential diagnosis in any situation where there is an inadequate explanation or concerning behaviours.
- Be clear of your facts, and obtain as much social history, including dates of birth and addresses, before discussing with social care.
- When exploring safeguarding issues, it is important to be aware of your limitations and seek a senior opinion whenever there is any doubt or uncertainty.
- Inform or update social care teams early in these situations.

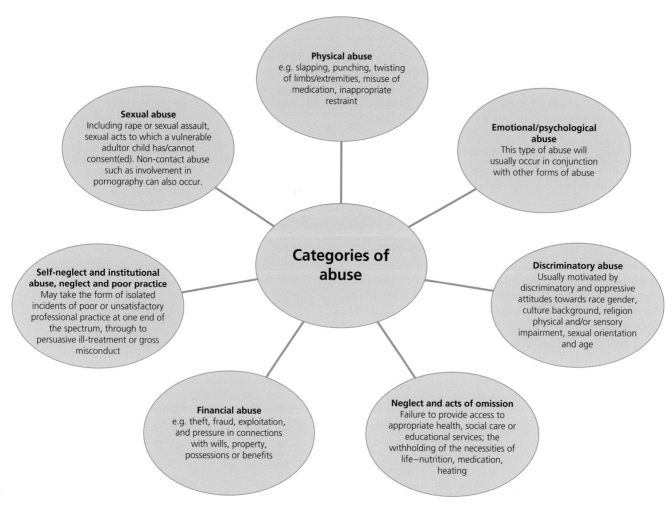

Figure 7.3 Common categories of abuse that require safeguarding actions.

- Be factual and non-accusatory with your terminology to the family – this is best explained using the case history in Box 7.3.

In this scenario, Peter the paediatric registrar remained calm. He was clear with the family that there were concerns about the injury and that it needed to be investigated. He remained clear about the process and which agencies would be involved.

In this situation it is important to allow periods of silence to permit a family to process the information, and allow time for questions and to check for understanding after you have summarised things.

Young people, risk-taking behaviours, consent and confidentiality

Consultations with young people (those aged 10–24 years) can be challenging for many reasons, including the following:
- During adolescence (10–19 years) there are physical, cognitive and socio-emotional developmental stages that all impact on effective communication with those around them, including health professionals who will need to adapt their approach.
- Young people usually want to feel listened to, have their concerns and opinions respected and be involved in their care, moving

away from reliance on their carers to becoming autonomous and responsible for their own health.
- Carers often want to be involved too, but young people should be given time to be seen alone for (at least part of) their consultations in order to identify any hidden agenda.
- It is important to assure confidentiality while also outlining its limits, e.g. when safeguarding concerns arise.
- Finally, the young person's jargon may need clarification to avoid embarrassing misunderstandings.

Consultations with young people may necessitate addressing physical, emotional and mental health, sexuality and relationships, body image, safeguarding concerns or risky behaviours. It is rewarding and vital to take a holistic approach to their care and the HEADSSS framework, outlined in Box 7.4, can be useful to ask some of the more difficult questions. Often, it is useful to 'normalise' behaviours with statements such as, 'Many young people try smoking around this time … is this something your friends have tried? What about you?' This can lead to more probing questions if necessary and relevant.

It is not always necessary to complete all the sections of the HEADSSS assessment at an initial meeting, and it is a good idea to start with a non-threatening section, bearing in mind that for some

Box 7.3 **Case history: safeguarding**

A young unmarried couple brought their 9-month-old boy in to the emergency department stating he could using his left arm properly. There was no clear history of an injury. A full examination of the undressed child revealed no bruises or concerning marks; however, there was swelling and pain in his upper left arm. An X-ray revealed a spiral fracture of the left humerus. The paediatric registrar, Peter, was asked to see the child and his parents.

Peter sat down and began by introducing himself and explaining his professional role. He clarified that the woman was the child's biological mother and the man her current boyfriend who has lived in the family home for 4 months. There were no other children in the home and no other children by other partners. Peter was mindful that the nature of his questions might make the couple feel anxious, angry or hostile. He therefore continued by confirming with them that there was no history of an accident or injury. He explained that the X-ray showed a broken arm. He asked again whether there could have been an accident or injury or any signs that the child may have been in pain or discomfort. He paused while the couple looked at each other. The child's mother burst into tears. Neither adult could think of a cause – he had been well, happy and playful until they had noticed he was not using his left arm that day. Peter explained that the injury was very significant and that, as there was no explanation for it, the normal thing to do in this situation was to investigate further.

The boy's mother looked very worried and asked if her child would be taken away from her. Her partner suggested that Peter was accusing them of hurting their child. Peter explained that he was not accusing anyone of injuring the child, but re-stated that when a significant injury has occurred with no explanation then it requires further investigation to try and establish the cause. Whenever a child has sustained an injury without an explanation, professionals are dutybound to follow a clear process that must be done without judgement, irrespective of the family's class, race or background. This does not imply any accusation towards anyone. Peter explained that his duty of care was to the child.

Peter further outlined that the process would involve medical tests as well as social services, the police and any other professionals involved in the care of the child, such as a health visitor. The mother and her partner became very quiet, but the mother said that she understood Peter's explanation and asked if her child was going to be okay.

Box 7.4 **HEADSSS framework for the psycho-social assessment of young people**

Home and relationships
Who lives at home with you? Do you have your own room? Who do you get on with best/fight with most? Who do you turn to when you're feeling down?

Education and employment
Are you in school/college at the moment? Which year are you in? What do you like the best/least at school/college? How are you doing at school? What do you want to do when you finish? Do you have friends at school? How do you get along with others at school? Do you work? How much?

Activities and hobbies
How do you spend your spare time? What do you do to relax? What kind of physical activities do you do?

At this stage – reassure about confidentiality

Drugs, alcohol and tobacco
Does anyone smoke at home? Lots of teenagers smoke. Have you been offered cigarettes? How many do you smoke each day? Many people start drinking alcohol as teenagers. Have you tried or been offered alcohol? How much/how often? Some young people use cannabis. Have you tried it? How much/how often? What about other drugs, such as ecstasy and cocaine?

If the teenager says yes to the above you should ask questions that assess their understanding of the harms/risks and their motivation to change their behaviour.

Sex and relationships
Are you seeing anyone at the moment? Are they a boy or girl? Young people are often starting to develop intimate relationships – how have you handled that part of your relationship? Have you ever had sex? What contraception do you use?

Self-harm, depression, suicide and self-image
How is life going in general? Are you worried about your weight? What do you do when you feel stressed? Do you ever feel sad and tearful? Have you ever felt so sad that life isn't worth living? Do you think about hurting or killing yourself? Have you ever tried to harm yourself?

Safety and abuse
It may not be necessary to ask every young person but it is important in those who self-harm, have established substance misuse or emotional/behavioural problems. Is anyone harming you? Is anyone interfering with you or making you do things that you don't want to?

Box 7.5 **Tips for improving communication with adolescents**

- Greet the young person and ask them to introduce those accompanying.
- Establish rapport with clear introductions, non-medical 'chat' and take their concerns seriously.
- Outline the concept of confidentiality (and its limits; see 'Further resources') clearly at the start of consultation.
- Remember the tasks of adolescence and adapt your style according to the young person's developmental stage – e.g. options for younger teenagers, open questions for older ones.
- Be non-judgmental and act as an advocate for the young person.
- Do not make assumptions – use gender-neutral terms until the young person's preferences become clear.
- Clarify teenage jargon you do not understand – don't try to be cool!
- Listen carefully and be genuinely interested in the young person.

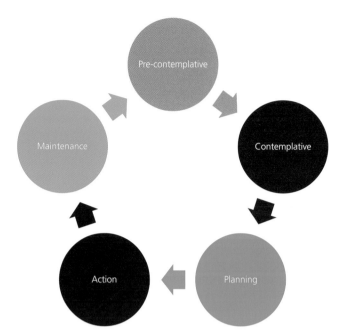

Figure 7.4 The cycle of change.

young people it may be particularly hard to talk about, for example, their home situation before rapport is built. Some tips for communicating with adolescents are outlined in Box 7.5.

Chronic disease

Given that adherence to treatment in acute illness can be poor, it is not surprising that compliance in chronic illness can be even more challenging. A patient with a chronic disease lives with that condition 24 hours a day, 7 days a week, 52 weeks a year, and the contact time with health professionals is a very small fraction of this. Patients may have to adhere to numerous medications, dietary restrictions, exercise and therapies, hospital visits and invasive investigations. Some regimens can be in conflict with living a 'normal' and relatively carefree life like everyone else. A grief reaction may be encountered not just at diagnosis, but at several stages along the way as control is lost. When confidence is low, inertia and inaction may result and it can be difficult to get back on track. Simply being told by health professionals what is good for you not only can be demotivating but can be completely overwhelming and cause resistance.

Motivational interviewing is a technique used to influence health behaviour through identifying factors that would motivate and effect change given the individual's life and unique set of circumstances by seeking the perceived benefits to the patient. Despite understanding why disease control would benefit them on a cognitive level, a change in behaviour only happens when an individual is motivated to want it to happen (see Figure 7.4). The challenge for a clinician is to identify personal motivators for change, to maximise these and minimise the barriers.

Boxes 7.6 and 7.7 outline the principles of motivational interviewing and give an example of a doctor–patient dialogue.

Seldom-heard groups

Seldom-heard groups are groups within a population who may have specific health needs (see Box 7.8) and who are difficult to engage in 'normal' health environments. Social services and many

Box 7.6 **Core principles and steps in motivational interviewing**

- Expressing empathy (establish rapport and understanding about how the situation is for the patient, how do they feel at the moment, normalise behaviour)
- Developing discrepancy (what is gap between how they think things are going now and how they would like them to be; what would be the motivators and benefits to change?)
- Resolving the patient's ambivalence (understand the conflict between the desire to change and the fear of changing and the barriers to enabling change)
- Supporting self-efficacy by emphasising autonomy (establishing self-confidence and self-belief in making changes)
- Rolling with resistance (as this is a signal that the patient views the situation from a different perspective)
- Avoiding argument (remain non-judgmental rather than viewing the patient as acting defiantly)

other organisations support such groups and can be involved in planning and establishing health services with them. Consideration should be made for how best to engage and communicate with these groups whose health needs are often unmet.

Conclusions

Advanced communication skills are sometimes required for specific situations and this chapter has given some examples: the triadic consultation; dealing with difficult behaviours; using interpreters; situations where there may be safeguarding issues; consultations with adolescents who are becoming more autonomous and may engage in risky behaviour, yet are still in some cases technically children; people who struggle with the demands of a chronic disease; and finally people from seldom-heard groups.

Box 7.7 **Example dialogue in a patient with chronic illness using motivational interviewing**

Dr Ahmed: I can see that you are finding blood testing difficult at school. I think this is true for most people. How do you think things are going?

Amy: I don't have time to check my bloods at school, only have 15 minutes for lunch as I'm going between one end of the building to the canteen which is at the other end.

Dr Ahmed: I imagine if you stopped to check your blood sugar, your friends may go and have lunch without you. Do you worry about that?

Amy: My friends don't know I have diabetes and I don't want to tell them. Yes, I'd rather not have lunch alone.

Dr Ahmed: How do you think they might behave if they knew about your diabetes?

Amy: Don't really know. I guess they'd probably be OK, but they'd ask a lot of questions.

Dr Ahmed: Are you worried their opinion of you might change?

Amy: No, I don't think so. I have good friends.

Dr Ahmed: I see. So you find it difficult when you are at school but easier when at home where you feel more comfortable and relaxed. It's really great that you are doing more testing at home, and this means you can correct high blood sugars and feel better in the evening when you have football training. I bet it improves your sports performance. Can you see any benefits to checking your blood sugar at school?

Amy: If I checked at lunchtime I could have a correction dose and I wouldn't be so tired in the afternoon.

Dr Ahmed: Why might this be a good thing?

Amy: I have exams coming up and I want to do well so I get my grades for next year, so it would be a good idea to check.

Dr Ahmed: I agree, checking your blood sugars would allow you to correct them to a normal range. This would mean your energy levels would be high, you would not be tired or thirsty or have blurred vision, and you might find it much easier to concentrate. On a scale of 1 to 10 where 1 is not at all confident and 10 is completely confident, how confident do you feel to start doing blood tests at lunchtime?

Amy: Probably 3.

Dr Ahmed: And on a scale of 1 to 10 where 10 is the most, how much would you like to have information on your lunchtime tests?

Amy: 8.

Dr Ahmed: That's quite a gap, Amy. How could we help you get from a 3 to an 8?

Amy: Not sure.

Dr Ahmed: Perhaps it is the fear of telling your friends about your diabetes which stops you? What do you think they might say?

Amy: They'd ask me lots of questions and I'm just not ready for that.

Dr Ahmed: I can understand that fear, but you might find that it's a big relief for someone to know what you are going through. Other young people have found it helpful to bring a close friend or partner along to clinic and they've said they feel happier when that person can ask the diabetes team questions instead. If you wanted to bring a close friend to clinic, that would be fine and we could help answer some of their questions here, with your permission.

Amy: I'll think about that. I might do.

Dr Ahmed: Is there any other reason why you find checking hard at lunchtime?

Amy: No.

Dr Ahmed: I see. Keep up the testing before and after school and let's revisit this next time.

Box 7.8 **Seldom-heard groups**

- Children in care and care leavers, particularly if multiple placements
- Travellers (i.e. people from the ethnic travelling community)
- Asylum-seekers
- People with sensory impairment
- Young carers
- Those with learning disability, reliant on carers to communicate
- Young people not in education, employment or training (NEETs)
- Young offenders
- Young people at risk of child sexual exploitation or trafficking, intimate partner violence, gangs and other safeguarding issues
- Lesbian, gay, bisexual or transgender individuals (LGBT)
- Families with strong cultural/religious beliefs.

Without a doubt, it takes time to develop good communication skills, and we often learn from experiences that have not gone so well. However, some simple approaches described in this chapter can be applied in certain situations to help make things go more smoothly.

Further resources

Department for Education. Working together to safeguard children: a guide to inter-agency working to safeguard and promote the welfare of children. March 2015. (Statutory guidance on inter-agency working). https://www.gov.uk/government/publications/working-together-to-safeguard-children--2 (Accessed January 2017).

Larcher V. Consent, competence and confidentiality. In: ABC of Adolescence. Viner R [Ed]. Wiley, Oxford. 2013.

Miller WR and Rollnick S. Motivational interviewing: helping people change. Guilford Press, 2012. www.motivationalinterviewing.org (Accessed January 2017).

CHAPTER 8

Communication and Mental Health

Lee Smith

Derbyshire Healthcare NHS Foundation Trust, Derby, UK

OVERVIEW

- Mental health problems are common in clinical practice and can pose specific communication challenges.
- The brief ordinary effective communication model emphasises that even brief encounters can have a large positive psychological impact.
- A person's story is key – understanding where people are coming from helps to put their behaviour in perspective.
- Encountering a patient with anxiety is probably the most common communication issue in clinical practice.
- There are some simple 'dos and don'ts' when communicating with people with delirium or dementia.

Introduction

Like all of medicine, our understanding of psychiatry and mental health is always changing. However, there is a lot of research that can help us to optimise our communication with people with mental illness. Mental health problems, whether they have an organic or psycho-social cause, are common and can have a significant adverse impact on people's lives. In some circumstances, communication can be difficult and this chapter outlines some of the ways we can communicate more effectively. Figure 8.1 illustrates the main areas that need to be considered. However, good communication is often based on everyday common-sense behaviours that we are all capable of – and these principles apply to *all* communication, not just when communicating with people with mental health problems.

Trust, respect and rapport

A key part of effective communication is the need for those present to feel the clinician is trustworthy and respectful. This requires building rapport. This is key if we want people in our care to feel safe, which in turn aids compliance with recommended treatment and recovery.

While in principle many clinicians are familiar with the concept of 'white coat syndrome' (the heightened anxiety that occurs while seeing a doctor), it is easy to forget the importance of this when working in a busy clinical environment. Many patients become passive or submissive in certain settings, or paradoxically agitated or aggressive due to their heightened anxiety and fear. Time taken to understand and apply basic counselling skills can benefit anyone struggling with mental distress – be it mild, moderate or severe; acute or chronic.

Many effective communication skills are common to our everyday experience and are things we appreciate ourselves. As a starting point, take a few minutes to consider how people have communicated with you in the past. What was it about their communication that was effective and put you at ease? Box 8.1 includes some of things that may have come to mind.

Brief ordinary effective communication

A lot of work on healthcare communication is counselling-based – it requires building a therapeutic relationship with someone and takes time. However, modern healthcare interactions do not usually have lots of time. Think about a 10-minute consultation with a general practitioner or ward nurses rushed off their feet in a busy general hospital. In mental health, the subject matter under discussion and the emotions expressed by the patient can be emotionally draining. No wonder it feels like we do not have the capacity to communicate effectively.

The brief ordinary effective (BOE) communication model, developed by Crawford *et al.* (2006), emphasises that even brief encounters can have a large positive psychological impact. It recognises the time constraints under which many health professionals work, and the emotional work required for many therapeutic encounters. In BOE communication there is an understanding that:

- Small talk ('phatic communication') is common in healthcare settings.
- Patients often do not want prolonged encounters.

ABC of Clinical Communication, First Edition. Edited by Nicola Cooper and John Frain.
© 2018 John Wiley & Sons Ltd. Published 2018 by John Wiley & Sons Ltd.

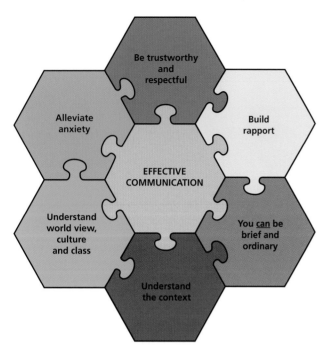

Figure 8.1 Effective communication in mental health – areas that need to be considered.

Box 8.1 Some things that characterise basic effective communication

- Introducing yourself by name – 'Hello, my name is…'
- Appropriate eye contact
- Appropriate tone of voice and body language
- A smile
- Good listening skills
- Being at the same level as the patient (e.g. sitting)
- Clarification of the content under discussion
- Affirming touch, where appropriate
- Storytelling or the use of analogy/metaphor
- Opportunity to discuss any concerns or possible misunderstandings
- Appropriate use of humour

- Brief encounters can leave their mark on people.
- Apparently ordinary encounters may mask more complex styles of communication.

People value and are comfortable with *ordinary* conversations – when there is some eye contact, a smile or a wave, small talk, non-medical language, and listening in turn. Brief and ordinary communication that is also effective takes into account the person's values and culture, it leaves the patient feeling satisfied and is linked to positive clinical outcomes.

For example, think about how you respond when you are busy in a clinical area and a patient or visitor approaches the desk to ask a question. If you work in a front-line speciality, how do you respond to patients queuing in the corridor or waiting room as you walk past? What is your body language like when you greet a new patient? How good are you at translating medical jargon in to terms people can easily understand?

Box 8.2 Brief ordinary effective (BOE) communication model in practice

A patient who had been admitted following an overdose of her antidepressant medication stated she wanted to leave hospital. A panicky message was passed on to the doctor: 'The lady in Bed 8 wants to take her own discharge. She's an overdose. She hasn't seen the mental health team yet. We might have to stop her from leaving. We're trying to get the mental health team to come now.'

The doctor went to see the patient.

'Hi, are you Sandra? My name is Nicola, I'm one of the doctors.' The doctor smiled, Sandra looked hesitant.

'Mind if I perch on here?' the doctor said, pointing to the end of the bed.

Noting that Sandra was a young English woman from a working-class background, the doctor sat down, looked at Sandra with a friendly face and said, 'You've had a bit of a crap day haven't you?'

Sandra grinned. 'Yeah,' she said. 'Tell me about it!'

The two had a conversation about why Sandra was so desperate to leave hospital before seeing the mental health team. It turned out her dogs were at home alone and she needed to get back to look after them. Sandra stayed to see the mental health team and then went home.

Of course, using such colloquial language is not appropriate for everyone. This same doctor would address an elderly patient by their surname and shake hands. Sometimes what is *ordinary* is hard to gauge at the beginning of a conversation. But this is an example of how ordinariness can be disarming.

Box 8.3 How one simple aspect of communication can improve patient satisfaction

Methods
A prospective, randomised, controlled trial was carried out on 120 postoperative in-patients who had been admitted for spinal surgery. The actual lengths of the interactions were compared with patients' estimations of the time of those interactions, and their satisfaction was also recorded.

Results
Patients perceived that the provider was present at their bedside longer when he sat, even though the actual time the physician spent at the bedside did not change significantly whether he sat or stood. Patients with whom the physician sat reported a more positive interaction and a better understanding of their condition.

Conclusions
Simply sitting instead of standing at a patient's bedside can have a significant impact on patient satisfaction, patient compliance and provider–patient rapport, all of which are known factors in decreased litigation, decreased lengths of stay, decreased costs and improved clinical outcomes.

Source: Swayden *et al.* (2012), abstract.

Box 8.2 gives an example of BOE communication in practice, and Box 8.3 describes how one simple aspect of communication can improve patient satisfaction.

Understanding the context

A primary part of any bio-psycho-social assessment is gathering and understanding the patient's story and context. Sound reasoning requires us to be able to acknowledge our own potential bias and lack of knowledge. There is a danger when communicating and assessing those with mental illness that we interpret what we see or hear through the limited lenses of our own understanding, without taking the time to clarify the situation further.

In fact, multiple factors need to be considered and can easily be missed if we are not prepared to take the time to understand the person's individual perspective. Examples include cultural practices, religious beliefs, sociological factors, relationship structures and support networks, and the impact of unresolved traumatic experiences, all of which can impact on the expression and mental and physical well-being of our patients. Some case histories illustrating unnecessary misunderstandings are given in the following sections. These are fictional but based on real cases.

Case history 1

A 30-year-old woman, recently arrived from India, was reviewed by her general practitioner for a routine pregnancy check-up. Her general practitioner was concerned because of reports that the patient spent most of the time sitting on the kitchen floor, rocking and chanting in her own language, seemingly in distress. He diagnosed a psychotic episode.

However, on further investigation, it turned out that this was a culturally acceptable practice in the region from which the woman originated. The rocking and chanting were, in fact, prayers for her unborn child. The woman was new to the UK, socially isolated and anxious. The initial diagnosis by a well-meaning but culturally unaware doctor was withdrawn.

Case history 2

A 65-year-old man was diagnosed with depression due to agitation and non-compliance with rehabilitation after several weeks in hospital. He appeared to be low in mood and resistant to physiotherapy interventions so he was referred to the mental health team.

Further enquiry revealed he was a farmer and spent the majority of his hours outdoors. It was lambing season, and he was concerned about how his farm was doing. He had no interest in television and had spent several weeks in a single room in hospital. He was being asked to manoeuvre into a chair hoist every day but no-one had explained why this was necessary or important and he felt unsafe in it, as if he might fall. When the patient's background and fear of the hoist were explained to the ward team, they were able to discuss his mood and fears and explain the importance of the rehabilitation process. Once this was done, his mood lifted, he complied with physiotherapy and was discharged a week later.

Case history 3

An 80-year-old woman with a long history of physical illness repeatedly expressed a wish to die. This alarmed the carers looking after her and she was referred for an assessment of her mental health. However, a simple conversation revealed that she had strongly held religious beliefs and was looking forward to a natural death when she would be at peace in a place called heaven. There was no evidence of suicidal intent or depression.

World view, culture and class

As you can see from the case histories in the preceding sections, the way in which different people view the world can vary enormously depending on their culture, social background and religious beliefs. This is often evident in their everyday perceptions and use of language. Even though all concerned in the case histories were living in the UK, people's world views can be very different.

A young person who says something is 'banging' means it is very good, whereas an older person is likely to use this term to refer to an intermittent noise. When an English student asks for a rubber they mean an eraser, but an American student is likely to be asking for a condom. In the same way, a person may appear to be highly agitated and paranoid during a conversation which – on the face of it – appears to be evidence of a psychosis. But if they are a gang member who is in trouble, there may be good reasons for their 'paranoia'. These examples illustrate how easily language and perception can vary despite us all speaking the same language. All these factors can impact on our communication with and understanding of people with mental health problems if we are not aware of them and do not seek to explore things further.

Understanding where someone is coming from is important in interpreting their behaviour. Figure 8.2 illustrates the factors that impact on communication and assessment of mental health.

Identifying and alleviating anxiety

Encountering a patient with anxiety is probably the most common communication issue in clinical practice. There are many causes of anxiety but, as well as normal 'worry', some of the most common are described in the following.

Unmet expectations. Everyone engaging in health services has a level of expectation about the service they expect, the way they will be treated by staff, and the care they will receive. If what to expect is not explained in the first place or not delivered, patients and/or their carers can become anxious, agitated or even angry because of frustration or fear. Examples of unspoken expectations that may be held with regard to different roles are illustrated in Figure 8.3.

Anxious attachment style. The ability to bond in relationships starts primarily in childhood. When a child has a secure bond with its parents then any feelings associated with anxiety or stressful situations can be alleviated in the presence of a safe caregiver. However, if the parent or caregiver is inconsistent, punitive or fails to reassure or comfort a child on a regular basis then ambivalent or avoidant responses to future caregivers may become entrenched in a person's relationship style in order to protect themselves from further emotional pain and rejection.

Threat/hypervigilance/unresolved trauma. People who have experienced or are experiencing significant trauma or threats (e.g. rape or domestic violence or other forms of abuse) often

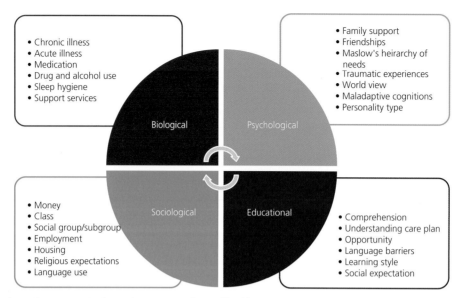

Figure 8.2 Some factors impacting communication and assessment of mental health.

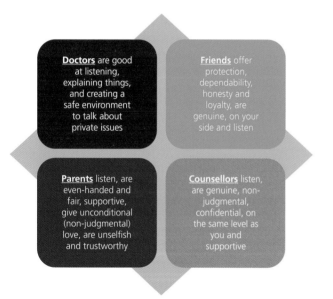

Figure 8.3 Unspoken expectations of different roles.

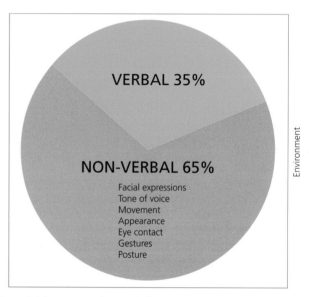

Figure 8.4 Importance of non-verbal communication. Non-verbal communication accounts for most of our communication, and also has cultural meaning. The environment in which communication takes place also has an impact on the effectiveness of communication. '*The most important thing in communication is to hear what is not being said*' (Peter F. Drucker).

develop 'hypervigilance' as a protective response. In some people this becomes ingrained and results in inappropriate physiological and mental responses or behaviours in unthreatening environments. For example, people with personality disorders often come from traumatic backgrounds and can respond with inappropriate aggression to perceived slights.

Medication. Sometimes anxiety can be triggered by new medications, interactions or polypharmacy. A 30-year-old woman was put on regular metoclopramide in hospital for nausea. She developed uncharacteristic restlessness and agitation which she could not explain. These are recognised side-effects of metoclopramide. Other examples include, but are not limited to, corticosteroids, regular cyclizine (especially in older people) and stopping antidepressants or sedatives abruptly.

Medical causes. Some anxiety or agitation is caused by medical problems but these may be missed. Hyperthyroidism, dementia, excess caffeine intake, recreational drug use, breathlessness, insomnia and alcohol withdrawal are examples. Sometimes treatment of an underlying medical condition will alleviate what on the surface appears to be a mental health problem. Unpacking any underlying medical problem requires good history-taking skills.

When seeking to alleviate anxiety and distress in a patient, clear communication is key. The environment, tone of voice, body language, content and timing of delivery is all important in de-escalating distress (see Figure 8.4). It is always worth reflecting on the fact that the same word can be used but delivered with a different emphasis or tone of voice and, as a consequence, can be interpreted very differently. Similarly, stressful/chaotic and busy environments (such as emergency departments) will usually escalate anxious and stressful feelings, but calm environments help to reduce them.

In all of the above, psycho-education (explaining where the feelings are coming from), reassurance and the normalisation of common experiences can help to calm a person's distress. Finally, it is worth remembering that the use of psychotropic medication can help, but the best long-term results are often achieved through a combination of counselling and medication, if required.

Resolving conflict in communication

The need to communicate with patients who are in some kind of mental or emotional distress is a common occurrence in clinical practice. Emotional distress can manifest as anger and frustration, or avoidance, passivity and non-compliance. There may be pressure of speech, or passive-aggressive communication (see Box 8.4). There may be delusions, hallucinations or other psychotic features. Common feelings underlying these presentations can be hopelessness, fear, anxiety, loneliness, bewilderment, lack of control, loss/grief, disbelief or numbness. Understanding this can sometimes help us to respond compassionately to the patient's needs.

The way people enter conflict varies, but common styles include:
- *Angry or competitive style* – manifests in a forcefully assertive stance, usually operating from a position of power, drawn from things like position, expertise or persuasive ability.

Box 8.4 **Passive-aggressive communication**

Passive-aggressive behaviour takes many forms but can generally be described as a kind of non-verbal aggression. Instead of communicating honestly when a person feels upset, they may display the following behaviours:
- Non-communication – when there is clearly something problematic to discuss
- Obstructing – deliberately stalling or preventing an event or process of change
- Ambiguity – being cryptic, unclear, not fully engaging in conversations
- Sulking – being silent and resentful in order to get attention or sympathy
- Making excuses – always coming up with reasons for not doing things
- Victimisation – unable to look at their own part in a situation to become the victim and will behave like one
- Self-pity – the poor me scenario
- Blaming others for situations rather than being able to take responsibility for their own actions

Passive aggression can be seen as a defence mechanism that people use to protect themselves, learned from early experiences as a form of avoidant behaviour. However, it is a very destructive form of communication.

- *Co-operative style* – seeks to meet the needs of all people involved. People with this style acknowledge that everyone is important and will seek to steer negotiations accordingly. If a variety of viewpoints are present then this style of communication is helpful in helping people reach informed decisions without compromising crucial facts.
- *Compromising style* – tries to find a solution that will partly satisfy everyone. All parties are expected to part with something of importance, but all are expected to gain from the negotiations. This can be helpful when the implication of ongoing conflict is worse than the benefit of ground gained.
- *Accommodating style* – exhibits a disposition to meet the needs of others if doing so is for a greater good. The accommodator can be encouraged to relinquish a position even when it is not warranted, often when the issues or ethical values matter more than a party winning or losing. Overall this approach is unlikely to achieve the best outcomes.
- *Avoidance and passive style* – seeks to evade the conflict entirely. People who adopt this style of negotiation are often fearful of hurting the feelings of others, avoid accepting roles in problem-solving, delegate contentious issues and negate key facts. It can be applicable when issues under discussion are inconsequential or beyond resolve, but for the majority of situations this is an ineffective approach to take.

Not all conflict can be resolved, but effective conflict resolution can be aided by the following:
- Listen very carefully to the concerns of the person – taking time to understand in the present can help to improve treatment in the future.
- Ensure you value the person's concerns and not just your own agenda – people 'catch' what you are, not only what you say. If you are genuine they will see and/or sense it; if not they will become defensive.
- Speak clearly and calmly in ways the person understands – use everyday illustrations if needed. Remember that people from different cultures, class or educational abilities may interpret what you mean differently from what you intend.
- Explain things – when people understand the reasons for treatment and have their concerns addressed, they are more likely to comply. Explore the pros and cons of decisions together to empower the person.

Communication in dementia and delirium

It is estimated that between one-third and one-half of hospital inpatients experience delirium, and with an ageing population, healthcare professionals increasingly find themselves caring for people with dementia. People with hyperactive delirium and dementia can exhibit challenging behaviour. It is important to understand that their behaviour can be made worse by things like medication, sensory deprivation, how we communicate and their environment. To help a person function at their best, all these areas should be optimised (see Figure 8.5).

For example, it is common to see relatives and healthcare professionals correct disorientated patients, or try to corral them back to their bed space. This usually has the effect of increasing agitation

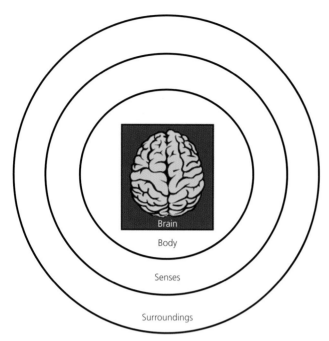

Figure 8.5 The interaction between dementia and the body, senses and surroundings. An interactive model of dementia. For successful treatment, all these interacting aspects of a person's function should be considered. *Source*: Courtesy of Wattis J and Curran S. Dementia, 2009. Reproduced with permission of Wiley-Blackwell.

and making things worse. Instead, relatives, carers and healthcare professionals should use the following strategies:

- Stay calm.
- Talk to the person in short, simple sentences. Repeat things if necessary.
- Use gentle re-orientation – remind them of what is happening and how they are doing.
- Do not contradict, go along with things and use distraction instead (e.g. change the subject).
- Listen to them and reassure them.
- Make sure they have their glasses on and hearing aids in.
- Ensure the environment is calm, well lit, and with some objects that help to re-orientate the person.

Conclusions

Communication in mental health can be difficult, but there are some basic principles that apply to all communication that can make things much easier. Be respectful, build rapport, be *ordinary*; try to understand where the person is coming from; be aware of world view, culture and class differences which could lead you to completely misinterpret what is going on; and use simple techniques to alleviate anxiety. Be aware that your body language speaks far louder than words; keep calm and explain things in simple terms; listen, don't contradict. Try to ensure your communication is happening in an environment that makes it easy to communicate and concentrate.

Most of the time, how *you* behave makes the interaction go smoothly. Sometimes however, in severe cases of agitation and distress, or even aggression, effective communication is impossible, no matter what you do. Do not see this as a failure. Remove yourself calmly from an aggressive situation. People need to be able to receive communication as well as give it, and, if they cannot, then leave it for another time.

References

Crawford P, Brown B, Bonham P. Communication in Clinical Settings. Nelson Thornes, 2006.

Swayden KJ, Anderson KK, Connelly LM *et al*. Effect of sitting vs. standing on perception of provider time at bedside: a pilot study. Patient Educ Couns 2012; 86(2): 166–171.

Wattis J, Curran S. Dementia. In: Cooper N, Forrest K, Mulley G, eds. ABC of Geriatric Medicine. Wiley-Blackwell, 2009.

Further resources

Gilbert P. The Compassionate Mind (Compassion Focused Therapy). London, UK: Constable & Robinson, 2010.

Oyebode F. Sims' Symptoms in the Mind, 5th edn. Edinburgh, UK: Saunders, 2014.

Sandars P. First Steps in Counselling, 4th edn. Ross-on-Wye, UK: PCCS Books, 2011.

CHAPTER 9

Communication at the End of Life

Adam Walczak[1], Phyllis Butow[2] and Josephine Clayton[2,3]

[1]CanTeen Australia, Sydney, Australia
[2]University of Sydney, Sydney, Australia
[3]Greenwich Hospital, Greenwich, Sydney, Australia

OVERVIEW

- There is no 'one size fits all' approach that will work for all patients and their families, but healthcare professionals should aim to have end-of-life discussions early enough that the patient can still be actively involved in their care and make appropriate decisions.

- Preparing for a planned end-of-life discussion is important to ensure optimal outcomes. However, it is important to acknowledge that patients or caregivers may initiate an end-of-life discussion at any point and thorough planning may not always be possible.

- Referral to palliative care services may evoke fears of impending death, helplessness and abandonment in the patient if the healthcare team does not communicate about this transition sensitively and effectively.

- Discussion of prognosis in terms that acknowledge uncertainty and present a range of potential outcomes is related to patients choosing less aggressive treatment options towards the end of life.

- When discussing cardiopulmonary resuscitation (CPR), an important consideration is ensuring patients and/or caregivers are aware of the poor success rate of CPR in patients with a life-limiting condition. When made aware this, they are less likely to choose CPR.

- Advance care planning is a *process* focussed on discussion, documentation and review of a patient's wishes for medical and other care in the future if they are no longer able to be involved in the discussion.

Introduction

End-of-life communication is challenging, in terms of both the skills required and the emotional impact on all involved. The need to deliver complex information, to balance realism with hope, communicate uncertainty and also convey non-abandonment pervades such discussions. Healthcare professionals often express uncertainty regarding how much patients want to know, or fear that they may lose hope if a poor prognosis is conveyed. Indeed, there are indications that clinicians often misjudge patients' preferences for information and their level of understanding. Consequently, patients are often not given the information they need to understand their prognosis and make informed choices.

A complex set of general and specific skills and knowledge are needed in this context. These include skills such as delivering bad news and acknowledging emotion. Helpful principles for undertaking these communication tasks are summarised in Figures 9.1 and 9.2 and further resources are listed at the end of this chapter. More specific skills include discussing palliative care, conveying a prognosis and its meaning, advance care planning and discussing cardiopulmonary resuscitation (CPR). These will be the focus of this chapter.

Timing of end-of-life communication

An overarching challenge for all parties approaching end-of-life communication is the issue of appropriate timing. It can be challenging to determine the point at which the end-of-life begins and thus when related communication becomes appropriate, with much variation depending on the illness and clinical context. There is broad agreement in research literature that once a disease is clearly not going to be cured and will be life limiting, end-of life communication is required. Elements such as communication about life expectancy, advance care planning and discussion of what is important to the patient are relevant to clinical communication even when a curative outcome is still possible, to inform decision making about treatment.

Some studies support the idea of having end-of-life discussions as early as possible in the illness, with indications that this is in line with patient preferences. Certainly studies suggest that many older and chronically ill patients welcome the opportunity to participate in advance care planning regardless of their prognosis. Other studies suggest that early discussions about end-of-life issues, such as at the time of diagnosis of a life limiting illness, can be distressing or that the information can be difficult to assimilate. Others still have

---

ABC of Clinical Communication, First Edition. Edited by Nicola Cooper and John Frain.
© 2018 John Wiley & Sons Ltd. Published 2018 by John Wiley & Sons Ltd.

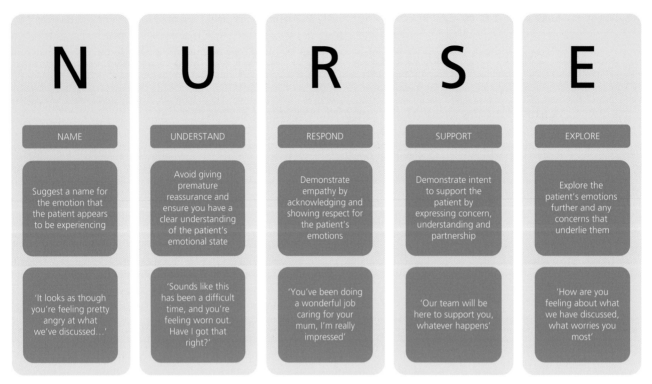

Figure 9.1 NURSE – a mnemonic to help accept, validate and acknowledge emotions and concerns. *Source*: Adapted from Pollack *et al.* (2007). Reproduced with permission of *Journal of Clinical Oncology*.

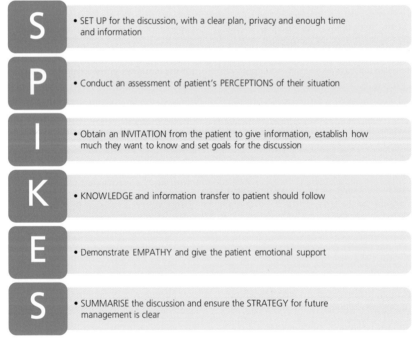

Figure 9.2 The SPIKES protocol for giving bad news. *Source*: Adapted from Baile *et al.* (2000).

identified patients' beliefs that the treating clinician should initiate these discussions using their common sense or intuition.

Overall, there is no 'one size fits all' approach, but given the potential for patients to experience cognitive and functional decline as their illness progresses, it may be important to have such discus-

sions early enough that the patient can still be actively involved in their care and make appropriate decisions about treatment, care planning or CPR with a realistic understanding of their situation, yet not so early that it causes undue distress. In addition, an early and routine introduction to the concept of advance care planning for all older or chronically ill adults may be another way to ensure all patients have the opportunity to discuss their wishes for care in case of a sudden deterioration in health.

Preparation for end-of-life discussions

Preparing for a planned discussion is important to ensure optimal outcomes. However, it is important to acknowledge that patients or caregivers may initiate an end-of-life discussion at any point in the illness, and thorough planning may not always be possible. Guidelines suggest that preparation should include reviewing the clinical records and speaking with relevant members of the clinical team to clarify the status of the disease and relevant comorbidities and gain up-to-date knowledge about the patient's underlying illness and treatment options.

It is also important to understand what the patient has been told by other healthcare professionals, such as their specialist or general practitioner, in order to provide consistent information. Allowing time to mentally prepare for the discussion may be important, particularly in the case of difficult or emotionally challenging patients, for example children or adolescents. Seeking advice from colleagues can also help to clarify how best to approach the discussion and learn from their experiences. Debriefing after the discussion can also be valuable, both as a learning tool and also to help with processing one's own emotions.

Empowering patients and caregivers

In the end-of-life setting, healthcare professionals often express great uncertainty about what patients want to know. Empowering patients and caregivers to express what information they want can greatly improve end-of-life communication. Patients often do not know what questions to ask. Many also do not know that discussing and documenting their preferences for end-of-life care is a possibility. They may be unaware of the appropriate time to ask about these issues or may delay initiating these discussions, believing that they have not reached a point in their illness where such issues need to be discussed. Patients may be concerned about being seen to be 'giving up' or may face overt resistance or discouragement from family members to openly discuss end-of-life issues. Likewise they may face an internal conflict between wanting to know about their prognosis and fearing bad news.

The following strategies may facilitate active involvement of patients and caregivers, and clarify their information and communication wishes:

- Communicating the possibility of discussing issues such as prognosis, advance care planning, not for CPR orders and your willingness to progress these discussions if the patient wishes to do so.
- Allowing time for questions and clarification and inviting patients and caregivers to contribute to the agenda at the beginning of the consultation.
- Providing tools such as 'question prompt lists' to help patients and caregivers ask questions. Several have been specifically developed for the end-of-life context (see Figure 9.3).
- Providing information and resources that may address patient/caregiver information needs and prompt further discussion.

Dealing with disparate information needs

End-of-life communication can be complicated by the presence of caregivers and family members in many consultations. As illness progresses, patients tend to want less information whilst caregivers often want more, particularly about future symptoms and disease progression. Caregivers may need more specific information than the patient about care needs as the illness progresses and how to get help if complications arise. This creates a challenge in negotiating and responding to different needs which may be in conflict. While there is an overriding need to respect the wishes of the patient

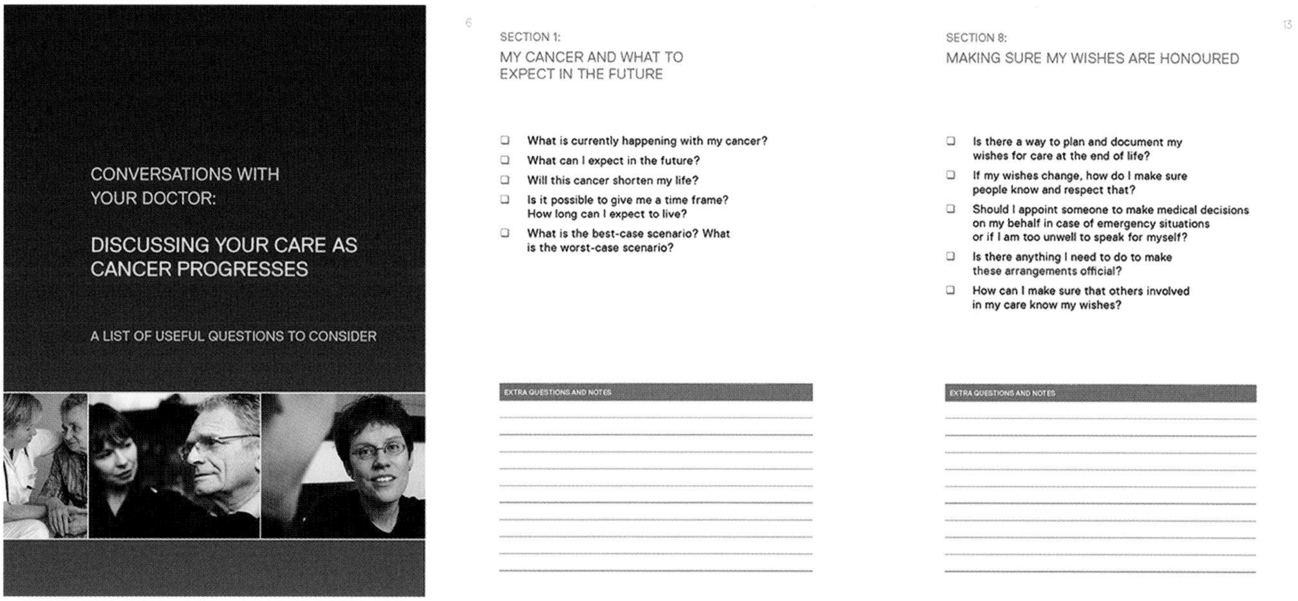

6

SECTION 1:
MY CANCER AND WHAT TO
EXPECT IN THE FUTURE

CONVERSATIONS WITH
YOUR DOCTOR:

DISCUSSING YOUR CARE AS
CANCER PROGRESSES

A LIST OF USEFUL QUESTIONS TO CONSIDER

- ☐ What is currently happening with my cancer?
- ☐ What can I expect in the future?
- ☐ Will this cancer shorten my life?
- ☐ Is it possible to give me a time frame? How long can I expect to live?
- ☐ What is the best-case scenario? What is the worst-case scenario?

EXTRA QUESTIONS AND NOTES

13

SECTION 8:
MAKING SURE MY WISHES ARE HONOURED

- ☐ Is there a way to plan and document my wishes for care at the end of life?
- ☐ If my wishes change, how do I make sure people know and respect that?
- ☐ Should I appoint someone to make medical decisions on my behalf in case of emergency situations or if I am too unwell to speak for myself?
- ☐ Is there anything I need to do to make these arrangements official?
- ☐ How can I make sure that others involved in my care know my wishes?

EXTRA QUESTIONS AND NOTES

Figure 9.3 Example 'question prompt list' questions – prognosis and end-of-life planning.

above all others, conflicting information needs can be addressed by having separate meetings with patient and caregivers if the patient is willing to give permission for this to happen.

Discussing palliative care

The World Health Organization defines palliative care as:

> An approach that improves the quality of life of patients and their families facing the problems associated with life-threatening illness, through the prevention and relief of suffering by means of early identification and impeccable assessment and treatment of pain and other problems, physical, psychosocial and spiritual.

However, the popular understanding of palliative care is that it focuses on care for those who are imminently dying. Referral to palliative care services may therefore evoke fear of impending death, helplessness and abandonment in the patient if the healthcare team does not communicate about the transition sensitively and effectively.

Key recommendations from clinical practice guidelines for end-of-life communication suggest introducing the palliative care team as part of the multidisciplinary team and clarifying patient and caregiver misconceptions. It may be useful to highlight that, compared with conventional disease-focused care, palliative care services provide better pain and symptom control, can reduce caregiver anxiety and increase the likelihood of the patient being cared for during the terminal phase in their place of choice. It may also be comforting for patients to know that palliative care can provide support for their family and children. Satisfaction with care is also likely to be higher.

Emphasising that the palliative care team can support the patient while they receive treatment for their underlying disease can address fears of abandonment. Reassuring patients that their primary care provider or treating specialist will still see them can also help to clarify the role of the palliative care team along with discussion of who they should contact regarding various issues or situations. An example of how to introduce the palliative care team is given in Box 9.1.

Discussing life expectancy

Although there is no clear evidence that one approach is better than another, various approaches can be used to communicate life expectancy estimates. These can include discussing the likelihood of being alive for a particular event (e.g. a birthday or graduation), giving a range of time (e.g. 6 months to a year), expressing prognosis in days, weeks or months (e.g. 'We're looking at weeks to months rather than many months'), or giving probabilities (e.g. 50% survival at 5 years). Some evidence from the cancer context suggests that giving the best-case, typical and worst-case scenarios can be a particularly good approach (see Box 9.2).

Patients may have an understanding of the uncertainty inherent in estimating life expectancy and value clinicians acknowledging this. There is good evidence that clinicians should avoid being exact with time frames unless in the final days of life, and there is some

---

Box 9.1 Example phrasing – introducing the palliative care team

'Part of the care we have on offer here is the palliative care team – they can provide extra support to you and your family to help manage things like pain or make sure you can get the most out of each day. We all work closely together to make sure you're as well as possible for as long as possible; I'll still be your main doctor and will still see you for some things, but the palliative care team will be able to provide extra support or advice with the best medicines for your pain.

'Most people have either never heard of palliative care or think that it's only for people who are dying in the near future. Have you heard the term before?'

[*following response*]

'How about we go through what you've told me and talk about what the palliative care team does... [*address misconceptions/concerns*]'

Box 9.2 Example phrasing – an option for giving a life expectancy estimate

'On average, patients with your type and stage of cancer live X months. One-quarter of patients will live Y months or less and one quarter live Z or more months. While I do not know for sure where you are in this group, the fact that you are feeling so poorly right now and in bed most of the time makes me concerned that you may not live longer than the average of X months.'

Source: Adapted from Lamont and Christakis (2003). Reproduced with permission of The JAMA Network.

---

evidence that patients prefer words or numbers rather than visual presentations. Discussion presented in terms that acknowledge uncertainty and present a range of potential outcomes is related to patients choosing less aggressive treatment options towards the end of life as well as improved patient understanding.

Advance care planning

Advance care planning is a *process* focused on discussion, documentation and review of a patient's wishes for medical and other care in the future if they are no longer able to be involved in the discussion. This is distinct from an advance directive, which is a written statement outlining a patient's wishes for future care. Completing an advance directive form and other important documents including substitute decision-maker or power of attorney forms are an important part of this process. Regardless of whether or not the patient chooses to complete formal advance care planning documents, participating in a discussion about advance care planning can improve care, particularly if the patient's preferred substitute decision-maker is also present. An example of introducing the topic of advance care planning is shown in Box 9.3.

Advance care planning helps patients to ensure they receive treatment and care that is in line with their preferences when they are no longer able to make decisions for themselves. It can help patients clarify their most important goals and priorities for care and facilitate open discussion between patients, their caregivers and clinicians about dying. Furthermore, it can reduce the burden on caregivers if they are asked to participate in treatment decisions on behalf of an incapacitated patient. Figure 9.4 illustrates the key steps in the advance care planning process.

Documented advance care plans or directives and substitute decision-making powers only come into effect once patients can no longer make their own decisions. Given this, it may be important to highlight that patients retain the right to make decisions for as long as they remain competent to do so.

Do not attempt CPR orders

An important component in end-of-life care is ensuring that CPR is not attempted inappropriately in someone who is dying. This is usually achieved by documenting a not-for-CPR order in the patient's medical records using an appropriate form. It is important to be aware of local guidelines and legal requirements when documenting not-for-CPR orders. Most guidelines recommend that CPR is discussed with patients and/or their substitute decision-maker and family, if the patient no longer has capacity to be involved, prior to completing a formal not-for-CPR order. This does not mean that CPR needs to be offered as a treatment option when the outcome is likely to be very poor. However, patients and families need to be prepared and know what to expect.

Ideally, discussion of medical orders for life-sustaining treatment, including CPR, should not take place in isolation but should be included as part of advanced care planning discussions along with broader discussion of prognosis, the patient's values, expectations and goals of care. Such discussions are often delayed until death is imminent, which can result in patients and families being ill prepared for death. Ideally a senior clinician with a good rapport with the patient should conduct these discussions well before the patient is imminently terminal.

When discussing CPR, an important consideration is ensuring patients and/or caregivers are aware of the poor success rate of CPR

> Box 9.3 **Example phrasing – explanation of the purpose of advance care planning**
>
> 'Have you ever talked about your wishes, values and beliefs about medical treatment and care in case you were ever injured or became too ill to speak for yourself?
>
> 'To help make sure your preferences are known, in case you are ever in this situation, there's a process we can go through called advance care planning. It can also help prepare you in case you need to make urgent healthcare decisions in the future, as it is often easier to talk through tough situations while you are still well.
>
> 'It's often best to include the right members of your family to make sure we all understand what's happening with your illness and what you want to happen. We also talk about who would make decisions for you if you couldn't, and write down the important things so everyone knows your preferences. It's also something we can discuss again if your preferences or something about your illness changes, so you're always in control.'

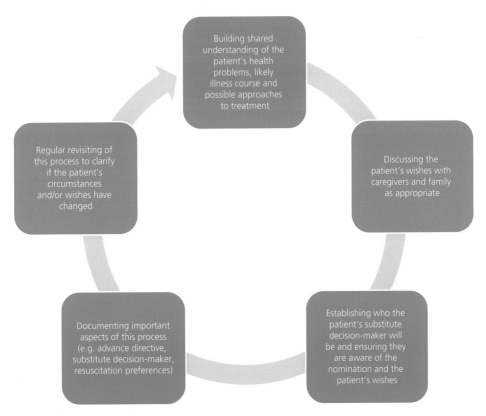

Figure 9.4 The key steps in the advance care planning process.

Box 9.4 **Example phrasing – explaining that CPR is unlikely to be successful and conveying non-abandonment**

'Cardiopulmonary resuscitation or CPR is given when a person's heart stops beating or breathing stops. It's used to keep people alive temporarily until they can receive emergency treatment in hospital or until an ambulance arrives. Given how advanced your illness is, trying to reverse that process and prolong life with CPR at that time is almost certainly not going to work and it could be distressing. Hence, I would not recommend attempting CPR.

'Not giving CPR does not mean that we are giving up on you. On the contrary, we will continue to be extremely active and supportive in caring for you. It simply means that when death does eventually come, our focus will be on keeping you comfortable and supported rather than prolonging the dying period. Allowing death to come naturally and making sure that you are as comfortable and supported as possible is our goal when that time comes. Is that in keeping with your thoughts and wishes?'

Or, *more briefly…*

'When the time comes I recommend allowing you to die naturally and doing everything we can to ensure you're as comfortable as possible. I recommend not attempting treatments like CPR that could cause distress and would not work in your situation.'

Source: Adapted from Clayton *et al.* (2007). Reproduced with permission of *Medical Journal of Australia*.

in patients with a life-limiting condition. It can be beneficial to explain that while most people think CPR is successful, the success rate in previously healthy people is actually fairly low and is *universally poor* in people with a serious progressive illness. When patients and families are made aware of these facts, they are less likely to request CPR. It is also important to emphasise that other care and support will continue to be provided. Box 9.4 gives an example of how to communicate this.

Conclusions

End-of-life communication is a particularly challenging facet of clinical communication requiring well-developed skills, confidence, knowledge and, perhaps most importantly, rapport with one's patient and their caregiver. Several training programmes have been developed to facilitate the acquisition of end-of-life communication skills, ranging from short workshops to multi-day residential programmes, several of which are listed in the 'Further resources' section. Opportunities to learn from the experience of colleagues, to debrief following end-of-life communication with patients and families, and to take a team-based approach to preparing for, practising and undertaking end-of-life communication are particularly valuable. Exploring and refining these skills within the safe context of clinical supervision and structured training programmes is highly recommended.

References

Baile WF, Buckman R, Lenzia R *et al*. SPIKES – A six-step protocol for delivering bad news: application to the patient with cancer. Oncologist 2000: 5(4); 302–311.

Clayton JM, Hancock KM, Butow PN *et al*. Clinical practice guidelines for communicating prognosis and end-of-life issues with adults in the advanced stages of a life-limiting illness, and their caregivers. Med J Aust 2007; 186(12 Suppl): S77, S79, S83–108.

Lamont EB, Christakis NA. Complexities in prognostication in advanced cancer: "To help them live their lives the way they want to". J Am Med Assoc 2003; 290: 98–104.

Pollack KI, Arnold RM, Jeffreys AS *et al*. Oncologist communication about emotion during visits with patients with advanced cancer. J Clin Oncol 2007; 25(36): 5748–5752.

Further resources

Back AL, Arnold RM, Baile WF *et al*. Approaching difficult communication tasks in Oncology. CA Cancer J Clin 2005: 55: 164–177.

Parker SM, Clayton JM, Hancock K *et al*. A systematic review of prognostic/end-of-life communication with adults in the advanced stages of a life-limiting illness: patient/caregiver preferences for the content, style, and timing of information. J Pain Symptom Manag 2007; 24(1): 81–93.

Steinhauser KE, Christakis NA, Clipp EC *et al*. Factors considered important at the end of life by patients, family physicians and other care providers. J Am Med Assoc 2000; 284: 2476–2482.

Walczak A, Butow PN, Davidson PM *et al*. Patient perspectives regarding communication about prognosis and end-of-life issues: how can it be optimised? Patient Educ Couns 2013; 90(3): 307–314.

CHAPTER 10

Teaching Clinical Communication

John Frain and Magdy Abdalla

University of Nottingham, Nottingham, UK

OVERVIEW

- Clinical communication is about deriving, recording and transferring high-quality clinical data about the patient as part of the process of clinical care. Teaching objectives should reflect this.

- The learning objectives in clinical communication teaching will vary according to the programme and the specific part of the curriculum.

- Learning objectives should be based on sound knowledge and theory in clinical communication skills. This should be apparent to the learner at each stage.

- Students should have the opportunity to observe, practise, give and receive feedback on their development in a non-threatening and supportive environment.

- There should be opportunity to display competence in oral, written and visual communication as well as using both verbal and non-verbal communication.

Introduction

In this chapter, we will describe an outline curriculum for clinical communication skills using the Calgary-Cambridge model of the medical interview (see Chapter 2). This model is used in 70% of medical schools in the UK and around the world. Our discussion reflects our own experience as teachers of clinical communication in a newly founded graduate entry medical school in the UK. Readers may wish to understand how the theoretical basis for teaching has been integrated with its actual delivery within a medical school curriculum. Resources covering the theoretical basis and evaluation of teaching are given at the end of the chapter.

During the first 18 months of their 4-year degree, our students study in a blended problem-based learning (PBL) course. This includes teaching in the basic medical sciences and a clinical skills course incorporating clinical communication teaching. In common with other medical courses, formal teaching of communication skills in our university is timetabled in the early years. At the end of the PBL course, our students start their clinical practice course, leading to qualification in the final year. Supplementing the pre-clinical clinical communication teaching are community and primary care placements which involve experiential, work-based learning on more advanced topics in communication skills, e.g. breaking bad news. Taken together, this curriculum reflects the topics covered in the UK Council's communication wheel (see Figure 2.2 in Chapter 2). The topics in the inner wheel form the basis of an introductory course (e.g. initiation and information-gathering), while those in the outer wheel contribute to a longitudinal curriculum with topics covered during the later clinical course and on placements such as primary or palliative care. However, the course is sufficiently flexible to allow topics from the outer wheel to emerge during pre-clinical sessions (e.g. presentation skills, talking to carers).

Engaging students

Having previously demonstrated good communication skills in previous degrees, careers and during the admissions process, there can be some reluctance among students to seemingly begin again to learn how to talk to people. Successful engagement needs sufficient motivation. This can sometimes be challenging if the students think that they already have these skills or if they simplify the concept of good communication to 'being nice' to patients.

It is important at the outset to assist students in appreciating the connection between good communication, particularly listening skills, and good clinical outcomes such as efficient use of time, better quality data from the history, improved diagnostic outcomes and patient compliance.

It is important for students to make the connection between a good history, responsible still for around 80% of diagnoses, and safe patient care. All students enter training wanting to be effective and accurate diagnosticians. It is essential that students understand how good quality clinical data (content) is derived best from good quality communication (process). As practising clinicians, we can

---

ABC of Clinical Communication, First Edition. Edited by Nicola Cooper and John Frain.
© 2018 John Wiley & Sons Ltd. Published 2018 by John Wiley & Sons Ltd.

Box 10.1 **Outline of video to illustrate quality of interaction using closed and open questions**

As an introduction to clinical communication training, two faculty members participate in a filmed conversation between two friends. This is shown to the students. Jo has just returned from a holiday. Anna asks Jo about her holiday. The film is unscripted, with Anna being instructed to ask only closed questions, 'What time was your flight?', 'What sort of plane was it?' in the first version, followed by open questions in a second filmed conversation on the same scenario. Later in each conversation Jo relates that she has returned home to find a family member is unwell. On both occasions the conversation proceeds to its natural close. After viewing both versions, students are invited to comment on the interaction between Jo and Anna in each conversation.

Commonly identified themes each year by students include:

- There are 44 closed questions in the first version versus seven open questions in the second.
- More detail emerges in the second version.
- Jo is more relaxed and there is greater rapport with Anna in the second version.
- Anna's body language displays greater empathy in the second version.
- Anna interrupts Jo less often in the second version.
- Jo can give more detail and express her concerns more openly in the second conversation.

The video enables us to illustrate the benefits of listening and allowing Jo to express herself in her own words and the shortcomings of list-like approaches to interviewing.

illustrate this with examples, positive and negative, from our own practice.

One area we have addressed at an early stage of engagement is moving students away from the concept of needing to know what questions to ask patients. This may be facilitated by promoting the idea of the medical interview as a conversation between friends. One would not converse with a friend using only closed 'yes' or 'no' questions, yet this approach characterises traditional history-taking. We have developed a video for students to illustrate the shortcomings of this approach (see Box 10.1).

In summary, giving students the evidence underpinning the process in eliciting good content is an important longitudinal theme in a clinical communication curriculum. This needs to be emphasised within the teaching sessions themselves and to be reflected also in other sessions within the clinical skills course (e.g. bedside teaching).

Clinical communication is teachable

Having established in students' minds that good communication skills are identifiable from research, and related to improved clinical outcomes, a subsequent step is to establish that these skills can be taught. Students vary in their personal (inherited) skills, which may make some more talented in communication. However, the communication skills of all can be improved through appropriate teaching. This requires:

- A suitable framework or model in which to situate the skills required in a medical interview.
- The identification and demonstration to students of the skills used in all consultations.
- The opportunity for students to practise or observe skills being used in a session.
- The opportunity for students to observe longitudinal development of both their own skills and those of others over time.
- The opportunity to receive feedback on their skills from patients, peers and teachers.
- The opportunity to rehearse and re-run aspects of interviews and skills.
- The opportunity for students to observe and use skills in the workplace through bedside teaching sessions or during early clinical experience attachments.

Longitudinally, a core set of skills may be required to be demonstrated (e.g. a checklist) but the whole should be coherent and capable of competently acquiring the biomedical data and patient's perspective necessary for the interview to be successful (i.e. globally proficient). This forms also the basis for assessment. With formative and summative assessment, students can progress in their learning and training. Performance outcomes in assessment can also assist in improving teaching methods.

Planning a curriculum – choosing a model

Several models for the consultation have been developed. Some are summarised in Box 10.2. Consultation models are not rules; they are learning aids to help learners develop their own consultation skills. Wise advice in using consultation models is to read them all, see which you like and take the best out of each to develop your own model. Good advice is also to have a range of different techniques to use in different and difficult consultations.

Our course employs the Calgary-Cambridge model as its starting point (see Chapter 2). It is well established in the UK. It utilises the evidence base for skills identified from research. Students progressing from pre-clinical to clinical placements will encounter clinical teachers in both primary and secondary care who were themselves taught using this model. There is therefore opportunity for role-modelling and reinforcement of skills within the real world of clinical practice.

Calgary-Cambridge is straightforward to explain to students, with its identification of phases within the consultation and discrete skills within each phase. While students may be initially daunted by the myriad identifiable skills within the model, many of the skills are inter-related and derivative of one another. In addition, clearly not every skill is needed on every occasion. Rather we are equipping them with a 'set of tools' for a variety of clinical encounters.

The model also provides an observation guide which provides both a checklist of skills and an aide memoire for students to generate feedback for the interviewer following a consultation. We have adapted the guide also to allow students and teachers to feedback on aspects of clinical reasoning and differential diagnosis (see Box 10.3).

Box 10.2 **Summary of common consultation models used in different curricula in North America and the UK**

Hermann's folk model, 1981
This model sees the consultation entirely from the patient's perspective using a series of questions such as: 'What has happened?' and 'Why me?'
  This model centres on the patient's story using empathy to address the patient's questions. Empathy is first recognising the patient's distress and secondly expressing the empathy. Statements to demonstrate empathy include: 'I can see how sad/frustrated/angry/frightened/upset you are.'

Pendleton *et al.* (1984)
This seven-task patient-centred model consists of defining the patient's true agenda, considering other problems, choosing an appropriate action for each problem, achieving a shared understanding, using time and resources appropriately and establishing and maintaining a relationship with the patient.
- Pendleton advises drawing out whether there are any other problems early in the consultation.
- This model introduced the concept of eliciting the patient's ideas, concerns and expectations.

Questions to try include: 'Was there anything else you were hoping to discuss today?', 'What is your main fear/worry/concern about this problem?' and 'What were you hoping to get out of today?'

Neighbour (The Inner Consultation) (1987)
This uses the five checkpoints of connecting, summarising, handing over, safety netting and housekeeping alongside an awareness of 'minimal cues' (verbal and non-verbal) to help discover the unspoken agenda.

Calgary-Cambridge guide (Kurtz & Silverman, 1996)
This model looks at the process of the consultation from initiating the session, gathering information, providing structure to the consultation, building a relationship, giving information by explanation and planning, and closing the session.

Defining the sessions – what needs to be taught?

As identified in the Calgary-Cambridge model, communication skills can be broadly divided into three categories: content skills, process skills and perceptual skills (see Chapter 2):

1 Content skills – what healthcare professionals communicate, i.e. the substance of their questions and responses.
2 Process skills – how they do it.
3 Perceptual skills – what they are thinking and feeling.

An overall aim is that students should enter their clinical placements with a framework of skills within which they can interview patients, begin to reason, and develop ideas about patient problem lists and differential diagnosis. Even from the initial stages of the course, students will encounter patients on early clinical experience visits or in bedside teaching sessions whom they will see interviewed or interview themselves. Indeed, these are positive learning moments as they will see skills role-modelled or otherwise and appreciate the application of these skills in clinical practice.

Among other objectives, students should know how to introduce themselves properly, including an appropriate definition of their role and stage of learning, obtain the patient's consent to interview, initiate and maintain a rapport, know how to make meaningful eye contact, how to start and maintain conversations, how to interact with all kinds of people, how to undertake a successful interview, manage relationships and eventually address the patient problem(s) with confidence.

Students must learn how to create rapport, trust and respect. These are the basic components of nearly every affirmative human interaction and can be applied in medicine as well as in other aspect of life where communication between two human beings is needed. These values are reflected in the overarching concept of the Calgary-Cambridge model.

Over the 18-month pre-clinical course we have broken the overall set of skills into manageable phases. These phases allow students to learn discrete skills, but also to incrementally develop their understanding of the model overall. Together these provide a robust framework for interviewing patients and obtaining a history during the clinical phase.

We have defined the following sessions:
- The opening statement
- Open questions
- Closed questions
- Process and content
- Background information
- The sexual history
- Using the medical record
- Focused history-taking.

Taken together these skills provide students with an outline for a complete medical interview into which students may bring other skills identified by the model (e.g. signposting, summarising). Box 10.4 summarises the content of these sessions, the subsidiary skills covered and the supporting evidence highlighted to the students. Further sessions cover additional themes:
- Feedback
- Listening skills
- Helping people change
- Explaining skills.

Each 90-minute session begins with a brief introduction on the skill to be covered, including, where appropriate, a short video demonstrating the skill. Students work in groups with a teacher and patient simulator on a scenario for 30–40 minutes. We have developed scenarios for each skill using a case-creation template (see Box 10.5). The scenario details for the patient simulator and teacher, the role to be played, the setting, areas for the patient simulator to provide feedback to the student and suggestions for variation of the role

Box 10.3 Adapted Calgary-Cambridge observation guide

Initiating the session
1. Greets the patient
2. Introduces self
3. Demonstrates interest and respect
4. Identifies and confirms patient's problem list
5. Negotiates agenda

Gathering information
1. Encourages patient to tell story
2. Appropriately moves from open to closed questions
3. Listens attentively
4. Facilitates patient's verbal and non-verbal responses
5. Use concise, easily understood questions
6. Clarifies patient's statements
7. Establishes dates

Understanding the patient's perspective
1. Determines and acknowledges patient's ideas
2. Explores concerns
3. Determines patient's expectations
4. Encourages expression of feelings and thoughts
5. Picks up verbal and non-verbal clues

Structuring the consultation
1. Summarises at the end of a specific line of enquiry
2. Progresses using transitional statements
3. Structures in logical sequence
4. Attends to timing

Building relationship
1. Appropriate non-verbal behaviour
2. Reads or writes in a manner that does not interfere with dialogue
3. Accepts legitimacy of patient's views
4. Empathises with and supports patient
5. Deals sensitively with embarrassing and disturbing topics
6. Appears confident and relaxed
7. Shares thinking with patient when appropriate

Explaining and planning – closing the session
1. Gives explanation at appropriate times
2. Gives clear, well-organised information
3. Checks patient's understanding and acceptance
4. Encourages patient to discuss any additional points
5. Closes by summarising briefly

Clinical reasoning and differential diagnosis
1. Elucidates a problem list
2. Identifies items of present illness
3. Possible diagnoses listed
4. Provides supporting factors
5. Provides refuting factors

Source: Adapted from Kurtz *et al.* (2004). Reproduced with permission of CRC Press.

Box 10.4 Overview of clinical communication sessions and sample key learning points

Session title	Sample key learning point
Feedback	It is important that feedback is given in a non-threatening and supportive manner
The opening statement	An opening statement allows patients to identify a problem list and is time-efficient
Listening skills	Active listening will encourage the patient to talk and enhance the quality of clinical data gathered
Open questions	Open questions encourage a full, meaningful response using the patient's own knowledge of the subject
Closed questions	Raising additional topics allows the interviewer to exclude particular symptoms. This is important in differential diagnosis and planning treatment
Helping people change	Demonstrate application of 'stages of change' model in assessing a patient's readiness to change and negotiating and planning change
Process and content	Appreciate the link between process and content of the interview in developing clinical reasoning
Background information	Establish evidence for previous diagnoses and identify previously undisclosed disease
Explaining skills	Start to achieve a shared understanding incorporating the patient's perspective
The sexual history	Practise gathering information about sex; identify common mistakes and barriers
Using the medical record	Wait for pauses when reading the notes, and signpost the intention
Focused history-taking	Focused history-taking uses the same sequence of skills but is more judicious in exploring background information

Tutor groups

One of the benefits of the course is that the same staff, who are also clinicians, teach clinical, communication and professional skills to all students. We have developed a tutor group system, meaning five to six students always work with the same peer group and teacher in both clinical and communication skills throughout the 18 months of the PBL group. This allows teachers to observe and monitor the progress of individual students, giving appropriate feedback and support where necessary and ensuring also that students participate regularly in the exercises. Teaching the skills requires good communication with and between the students themselves, and their trust. Our system facilitates the development of a supportive learning environment within sessions which develops over time. Learning communication skills cannot be achieved in isolation. The students practise within their groups, having the chance of observing, giving and receiving feedback. Emphasis is placed on the student conducting an interview, providing raw material for discussion within the group. Subsequently, the complete interview or elements identified during feedback can be re-run by either the same or another student. By undertaking two scenarios within each session, each of the students should have an opportunity to interview, observe, give and receive feedback, summarise and present a history.

subject to how the session develops on the day. Scenarios are written for both primary and secondary care so that students may appreciate how skills can be used in relation to interviews undertaken in both settings. As the PBL course is a modular one, scenarios take account also of the current module so that, for example, the scenarios written for the 'open questions' session relate to presentations of respiratory symptoms.

Box 10.5 **Case-creation template for patient simulator roles – completed for introductory case (Division of Medical Sciences and Graduate Entry Medicine, University of Nottingham)**

Case author	John Frain
Date of writing	18 July 2015
Name of patient	Mr Patrick James
Purpose of case	• Introduce students to patient simulators
	• Establish purpose of ALOBA
	• Introduce students to following skills
	○ Introduction
	○ Clarification of role
	○ Establishing purpose of interview
	○ Taking an opening statement
	○ Identifying an agenda
	○ Summarising
	○ Closure
	○ Presentation
	○ Beginning of clinical reasoning
Learner's level of expertise	First-year medical students in Module 1
What sort of case is this?	Training
Anticipated length of interview	5–10 minutes maximum
Patient's problem	A red, swollen leg
Key challenges	Overcoming students' shyness and apprehensiveness
	Establishing a structure to the training
Differential diagnosis	Cellulitis
	DVT
	Boil
	Insect bite
	Trauma
Setting	Hospital A&E department
Method of analysis	Calgary-Observation guide and ALOBA
Patient simulator to give feedback on	Did the student clarify who you were?
	Did the student clarify their role and the purpose of the interview?
	Were you able to give a description of your problem, including your concerns, before the student asked you any questions?
	Feedback on student's own agenda items

Feedback

Feedback can be used to enhance students' insight and reflections on the areas where improvement is needed, as well as highlighting and confirming good practice. Simulated patients, teachers and all students participate in feedback. The Calgary-Cambridge observation guide forms the mainstay for this process. It is initially necessary while students find their feet in giving feedback that is detailed, specific and non-judgmental. In time, students learn to set their own objectives using the Agenda-Led Outcome Based Analysis (ALOBA) objectives.

Engagement can be achieved by the proper setting and explanation of objectives, explanation of the process of learning itself, and by setting relevant ground rules in the teaching session. Ground rules may involve the practical steps of running the session with clear allocation of the different tasks as well as stressing the basic principles like confidentiality, mutual respect and teamwork spirit.

Box 10.6 **Robert, second-year medical student**

'There are subtle skills about communicating with patients that you don't get to practise apart from with a patient simulator. That's why patient simulators are integral (to the clinical communication course). You can use those models and go in and start practising how you actually talk to someone; how you start to access their story. A normal conversation is fine, but there also stages in your head you have to build up. The patient simulators are integral to practising, so that when you start to talk to real patients you are precise and efficient at gaining access to the story and especially the most important clinical parts of that story.

'For me especially, I look forward to coming in to talk to the patient simulators. They are great actors. They give you a full story and it is very convincing. You really think about the presentation and because the presentations are clinical, not only are you able to practise communication skills, but in a sense it is actually a way of building a picture of what someone might actually present with in terms of their clinical history.'

An introductory session on feedback is given in which students interview one another within their tutor groups on a non-medical topic (e.g. what you did before you started this course, or over the summer). They use a form of the observation guide adapted for this purpose.

Role of simulated patients

Simulated patients emerged in the 1960s and are now commonplace in many healthcare education settings. Many simulated patients are from acting backgrounds. They are familiar with professionals at all levels of training. Well-trained simulated patients are as effective as real patients in being interviewed. They enable students to learn under safe supervision in an environment where mistakes can be made and reflection undertaken. The opportunity to re-run and rehearse consistently facilitates improvement in clinical communication skills. Supportive feedback also promotes development of self-awareness among students and facilitates the development of alternative strategies when interviewing different patients (see Box 10.6).

Marrying process and content

An identified shortcoming of communication skills courses is the difficulty of teaching process and content alongside one another in a manner reflective of real-world clinical practice. We have addressed this by running sessions parallel to the communication skills session in which students consider strategies for identifying the relevant content of the patient's history in terms of clinical data. These 'exploring symptoms' sessions consider the anatomical and physiological basis of symptoms, the words patients use to describe them and the epidemiological evidence for the significance of symptoms, as we wish to promote Osler's maxim, 'Listen to the patient; he is telling you the diagnosis.'

There is a risk in the 'exploring symptoms' sessions of promoting lists of questions to be asked of patients. This is addressed using trigger videos from websites such as www.healthtalk.org, where students listen to patients describing their experience of a condition. For example, when considering cardiac chest pain, students watch four videos of patients describing their pain and then discuss the common elements of these four different stories which suggest cardiac rather than other causes of chest pain. The groups move on to discuss strategies for gathering key content relating to symptoms within the cardiovascular symptom using their listening and other communication skills.

A further opportunity for marrying process and content is provided at 'bedside teaching' sessions. These are attended by patients with conditions relevant to the current module of study. Students again learn within the tutor group with their teacher. One student interviews the patient whilst peers and teacher observe and feedback on both the process and content of the interview. For this purpose, we have developed an additional observation guide, which includes a summarised version of the Calgary-Cambridge observation guide, but includes also descriptors for the content of the interview (see Box 10.7). The patient is also invited to give feedback on the experience of being interviewed by individual students. Students can see and therefore begin to learn the balance between the process and content of eliciting a medical history.

Presentation skills

Both within and between healthcare teams, presentation and communication of patient information is essential for good care (see Chapter 5). For the student, the quality of a presentation may be the only evidence an assessor has for judging the quality of a history. As well as being an essential workplace skill, it is important for students to learn to do themselves justice in front of their teachers and to perform with confidence. Indeed, it is emphasised that the assessment of students' interviewing skills in clinical practice may more often be inferred from case presentations than from direct observation.

Also integrated within our teaching sessions is a requirement for the student conducting an interview to present their history to their tutor group and also to receive feedback on the process and content of their presentation. Students are provided with a sample grid to facilitate this (see Box 10.8).

This grid could be further adapted to include examination findings, a problem list and management plan.

Role of this model in experiential inter-professional learning

The current and well-documented difficulties in inter-professional communication (see Chapters 1 and 5) may be addressed in part by learning alongside one another. Doctors in many specialities work increasingly alongside advanced nurse practitioners and physicians' associates who utilise similar skills when communicating with patients and each other. This model provides the possibility of a supportive environment where health professionals can learn together.

Box 10.7 **Graduate Entry Medicine Observation Guide (Division of Medical Sciences and Graduate Entry Medicine, University of Nottingham)**

Communication and professionalism
1. Introduces self and checks patient's name
2. Clarifies own role
3. Obtains consent
4. Hand washing
5. Allows the patient to make an opening statement
6. Identifies a reason for the consultation
7. Continues with open questions to explore the presenting symptoms
8. Uses pertinent closed questions
9. Checks and summarises
10. Closes the consultation and 'hands over'

The presenting complaint
1. Is the presenting symptom(s) clearly identified?
2. Were appropriate descriptors used?
3. Were associated symptoms identified?
4. Is the sequence of events clear?
5. Is the level of detail appropriate?
6. Were relevant positives and negatives identified?

Review of symptoms
1. Was an appropriate review of symptoms performed?
2. Were any key relevant features missed?

Past medical/family/social history
1. Was the past medical history identified?
2. Were irrelevant events avoided?
3. Were items already presented in the presenting complaint left out?
4. Were all medications listed with generic names?
5. Were alternative and over-the-counter medicines listed?
6. Were allergies and the nature of the reaction included?
7. Was smoking/alcohol/substance misuse identified?
8. Were major medical issues in the family discussed?
9. Were relevant aspects of the social history included?

Physical examination
1. Did examination start with a description of the patient's physical appearance?
2. Were vital signs measured?
3. Did the examination follow a logical sequence?
4. Was the examination appropriate and detailed enough for the presenting complaint?
5. Was anything missing?

Differential diagnosis
1. A list of possible diagnoses is identified in descending order of likelihood
2. The conditions listed are relevant to the patient's age, sex, race and setting
3. The conditions listed are relevant to the patient's history and examination findings
4. The differential diagnosis is supported by clear reasoning

Summary
1. Was the presentation clear, concise and well organised?
2. Were summaries of both the history and presenting complaint presented?
3. The presentation was made with appropriate eye contact with the patient and the rest of the group
4. There was minimal use of notes as an aide-memoire

Box 10.8 **Presentation of the history template (Division of Medical Sciences and Graduate Entry Medicine, University of Nottingham)**

The presenting complaint
A brief description of your patient and his/her main symptom
'This is' **name, age, sex** 'who is a' **occupation** 'presenting with' **main presenting symptom**

History of the presenting complaint
'The problem first began when ......
- Describe onset, duration, variation of symptoms, exacerbating, relieving factors
- Effect on patient's life, occupation, social, family
- Associated features – accompanying symptoms or features, often within the same system, which may suggest particular disease
- Risk factors
- Relevant past medical history
- Patient's ideas and concerns about the problem

Review of systems

Past medical history
- Major diagnoses
- Medication – including allergies/intolerances
- Smoking/alcohol if not mentioned above
- Family and social history

Summary of the history (no more than two to three sentences)
'In summary, this is ... **name, age, sex, occupation,** who presents with **key presenting symptom(s)**. S/he is concerned about .... **effects on life, effects on health**'

Differential diagnosis
My differential diagnosis would be ......
1. .... because ....
2. .... because ....
3. .... because ....
4. .... because ....

Conclusions

Evidence-based clinical communication can by taught as a longitudinal theme within a pre-clinical clinical skills course (see Box 10.9). The skills and the model can be both taught separately and integrated with other themes such as history-taking and reasoning. Small group teaching with simulated patients assists with skills transfer to students, while bedside teaching and early clinical experience visits reinforce observation, practice and feedback on interviewing skills.

Box 10.9 **Robert, second-year medical student**

'When you first start medical school, you don't really have any appreciation of how important the history really is and you get told the history is the number one most important tool you have as a doctor. And you really develop this appreciation as the course goes on.'

Acknowledgements

We would like to acknowledge the help of Robert Armstrong, second-year medical student, for comments on the text and permitting us to use his words.

References

Kurtz S, Silverman J, Draper J. Teaching and Learning Communication Skills in Medicine, 2nd edn. CRC Press, 2004.

Kurtz S, Silverman J. Skills for Communicating with Patients. Oxford, UK: Radcliffe Medical Press, 1998.

Neighbour R. The Inner Consultation: How to Develop an Effective and Intuitive Consulting Style. Springer, 1987.

Pendleton D. The Consultation: An Approach to Learning and Teaching. Oxford General Practice Series, 1984.

Further resources

Del Mar C, Doust J, Glasziou PP. Clinical Thinking: Evidence, Communication and Decision-making. Oxford: BMJ Books. Oxford, 2006.

von Fragstein M, Silverman J, Cushing A et al. UK consensus statement on the content of communication curricula in undergraduate medical education. Med Educ 2008; 42 (11): 1100–1107.

Hargie O, Boohan M, McCoy M, Murphy P. Current trends in communication skills training in UK schools of medicine. Med Teacher 2010; 32(5): 385–391.

Keifenheim KE, Teufel M, Speiser N et al. Teaching history taking to medical students: a systematic review. BMC Med Educ 2015; 15: 159.

Silverman J, Kurtz SM, Draper J. Skills for Communicating with Patients, 3rd edn. Oxford, UK: Radcliffe, 2013.

Health Talk. Learning and Teaching. Online: www.healthtalk.org/learning-teaching. Accessed: May 2017. A useful website with patient histories useful for teaching and learning.

Recommended Books, Articles and Websites

For students and teachers

Brown J, Noble LM, Papageorgiou A, Kidd J. Clinical Communication in Medicine. Wiley, 2016.

Crawford P, Bonham P, Brown B. Foundations in Nursing and Health Care – Communication in Clinical Settings. Cengage Learning, 2006.

Del Mar C, Doust J, Glasziou P. Clinical Thinking: Evidence, Communication and Decision-making. BMJ Books, 2006.

Jackson C. Shut Up and Listen: a Brief Guide to Clinical Communication Skills. Dundee University Press, 2008.

Lloyd M, Bor R. Communication Skills for Medicine, 3rd edn. Churchill Livingstone, 2009.

Neighbour R. The Inner Consultation: How to develop an effective and intuitive consulting style, 2nd edn. CRC Press, 2015.

Tate P, Tate E. The Doctor's Communication Handbook, 7th edn. CRC Press, 2014.

Washer P. Clinical Communication Skills. Oxford University Press, 2009.

Academic

British Medical Association. Safe Handover, Safe Patients. Guidance on Clinical Handover for Clinicians and Managers. London, UK: British Medical Association, 2004.

Francis, R. Report of the Mid Staffordshire NHS Foundation Trust Public Inquiry: executive summary, Feb. 2013.

Kurtz S, Silverman J, Draper J. Teaching and Learning Communication Skills in Medicine, 2nd edn. CRC Press, 2004.

Pendleton D. The New Consultation: Developing Doctor-Patient Communication. Oxford University Press, 2003.

Silverman J, Kurtz S, Draper J. Skills for Communicating with Patients, 3rd edn. CRC Press, 2013.

Articles

Aspegren K, Lonberg-Masden P. Which basic communication skills in medicine are learnt spontaneously and which need to be learnt and trained? Med Teach 2005; 27(6): 539–543.

Barrett A. Evidence based medicine and shared decision making: the challenge of getting both evidence and preferences into health care. Patient Educ Couns 2008; 73: 407–412.

Bensing JM, Deuveugle M, Moretti F et al. How to make the medical consultation more successful from a patient's perspective? Tips for doctors and patients from lay people in the United Kingdom, Italy, Belgium and the Netherlands. Patient Educ Couns 2011; 84: 287–293.

Brown J. How clinical communication has become a core part of medical education in the UK. Med Educ 2008; 42: 271–278.

Car J, Sheikh A. Telephone consultations. Br Med J 2003; 326: 966–942.

Chewning B, Bylund CL, Shah B et al. Patient preferences for shared decisions: A systematic review. Patient Educ and Couns 2012; 86: 9–18.

De Haes H, Bensing J. Endpoints in medical communication research, proposing a framework of functions and outcomes. Patient Educ Couns 2009; 74(3): 287–294.

Elwyn G, Frosch D, Thomson R et al. Shared decision making: A model for clinical practice. J Gen Intern Med 2012; 27(10): 1361–1367.

Elwyn G, Laitner S, Coulter A et al. Implementing shared decision making in the NHS. Br Med J 2010; 14: 341

Fink AS, Prochazka AV, Henderson WG et al. Enhancement of surgical informed consent by addition of repeat back: A multicenter, randomised controlled clinical trial. Ann Surg 2010; 252: 27–36.

Frankel R, Stein T. Getting the most out of the clinical encounter: the four habits model. Permanente J 1999; 3(3): 79–88.

Hagerty RG, Butow PN, Ellis PA et al. Cancer patient preferences for communication of prognosis in the metastatic setting. J Clin Oncol 2004; 22: 1721–1730.

Hall JA. Clinicians' accuracy in perceiving patients: Its relevance for clinical practice and a narrative review of methods and correlates. Patient Educ Couns 2011; 84: 319–324.

Han PK, Jockes K, Elwyn G et al. Development and evaluation of a risk communication curriculum for medical students. Patient Educ Couns 2014; 94(1): 43–49.

Henry SG, Fuhrel-Forbis A, Rogers MAM, Eggly S. Association between nonverbal communication and outcomes: A systematic review and meta-analysis. Patient Educ Couns 2012; 86: 297–315.

Hudak PL, Armstrong K, Braddock C et al. Older patients' unexpressed concerns about orthopaedic surgery. J Bone Joint Surg 2008; 90: 1427–1435.

Joseph-Williams N, Elwyn G, Edwards A. Knowledge is not power for patients: A systematic review and thematic synthesis of patient-reported barriers and facilitators to shared decision making. Patient Educ Couns 2014; 94: 291–309.

ABC of Clinical Communication, First Edition. Edited by Nicola Cooper and John Frain.
© 2018 John Wiley & Sons Ltd. Published 2018 by John Wiley & Sons Ltd.

Kalet A, Pugnaire MP, Cole-Kelly K et al. Teaching communication in clinical clerkships: models from the Macy initiative in health communications. Acad Med 2004; 79(6): 511–520.

Kurtz S, Silverman J, Benson J, Draper J. Marrying content and process in clinical method teaching: Enhancing the Calgary-Cambridge guides. Acad Med 2003; 78(8) 802–809.

Langseth MS, Shepherd E, Thomson R, Lord S. Quality of decision making is related to decision outcome for patients with cardiac arrhythmia. Patient Educ Couns 2012; 87: 49–53.

Makoul G. The SEGUE Framework for teaching and assessing communication skills. Patient Educ Couns 2001; 45(1): 23–34.

Makoul G. Essential elements of communication in medical encounters: the Kalamazoo consensus statement. Acad Med 2001; 76(4) 390–393.

Montori VM, Shah ND, Pencille LJ et al. Use of a decision aid to improve treatment decisions in osteoporosis: the osteoporosis choice randomised trial. Am J Med 2011; 124(6): 549–556.

Shah S, Andrades M, Basir F et al. Has the inclusion of a longitudinally integrated communication skills program improved consultation skills in medical students? A pilot study. J Family Med Primary Care 2016; 5(1): 45–50.

Shepherd HL, Butow PN, Tattersall MHN. Factors which motivate cancer doctors to involve their patients in reaching treatment decisions. Patient Educ Couns 2011; 84: 229–235.

Shepherd HL, Barratt A, Trevena LJ et al. Three questions that patients can ask to improve the quality of information physicians give about treatment options: A cross-over trial. Patient Educ Couns 2011; 84: 379–385.

Simpson M, Buckman R, Stewart M et al. Doctor-patient communication: the Toronto consensus statement. Br Med J 1991; 303: 1385–1387.

Stacey D, Bennett CL, Barry MJ et al. Decision aids for people facing health treatment or screening decisions. Cochrane Database of Systematic Reviews, 10 (art no: CD001431).

Stewart MA. Effective physician-patient communication and health outcomes: a review. CMAJ 1995; 152(9):1423–1433.

Websites (all accessed January 2017)

Advance Care Planning Australia: http://advancecareplanning.org.au

Advance Care Planning: Tips from the National Institute on Aging: https://www.nia.nih.gov/health/publication/advance-care-planning

Cancer Network. Discussing Cancer Prognosis: http://www.cancernetwork.com/oncology-journal/discussing-cancer-prognosis

General Medical Council. *Treatment and Care Towards the End of Life: Good Practice in Decision Making*: http://www.gmc-uk.org/Treatment_and_care_towards_the_end_of_life___English_1015.pdf_48902105.pdf

http://www.ukccc.org.uk

Institute for Healthcare Communication. Conversations at the End of Life: http://healthcarecomm.org/training/continuing-education-workshops/conversations-at-the-end-of-life/

International Association for Communication in Healthcare: http://www.each.eu

Mayo Clinic Shared Decision Making National Resource Center: http://shareddecisions.mayoclinic.org

Option Grid decision aids: http://optiongrid.org

The Health Foundation. MAGIC: Shared Decision Making: http://www.health.org.uk/programmes/magic-shared-decision-making

UpToDate. Advance care planning and advance directives: http://www.uptodate.com/contents/advance-care-planning-and-advance-directives

VITAL Talk: http://www.vitaltalk.org

Index

ABC of Clinical Communication, First Edition. Edited by Nicola Cooper and John Frain.
© 2018 John Wiley & Sons Ltd. Published 2018 by John Wiley & Sons Ltd.

WITHDRAWN
FROM LIBRARY

BMA

BRITISH MEDICAL ASSOCIATION